Forgive
and
Remember

Charles L. Bosk

Forgive and Remember

Managing Medical Failure

Second Edition

The University of
Chicago Press
Chicago and London

The University of Chicago Press, Chicago 60637
The University of Chicago Press, Ltd., London
© 1979, 2003 by The University of Chicago
All rights reserved
Published 2003
Printed in the United States of America
12 11 10 09 08 07 06   2 3 4 5
ISBN: 0-226-06678-9 (paper)

Library of Congress Cataloging in Publication Data

Bosk, Charles L.
    Forgive and remember : managing medical failure /
Charles L. Bosk.—2nd ed.
        p. cm.
    Previously published in 1979.
    Includes bibliographical references and index.
    ISBN 0-226-06678-9 (pbk. : alk. paper)
    1. Surgery—Study and teaching (Graduate)—Social
aspects. 2. Surgical errors. 3. Surgery—Quality
control. 4. Surgeons. I. Title.
    RD28.A1B67 2003
    617—dc21   2003048352

To the memory of my
mother and father,
whose norms I cherish,
whose quasi-norms I
miss

Contents

Acknowledgments

Field work, like surgery, is a "body-contact" sport, and the surgeons at Pacific Hospital never shrank from this contact. In what were often very trying circumstances, they were considerate, candid, and courteous beyond the limits of any social and academic obligation. If they taught me nothing else, the surgeons taught me that delivering high-quality humane care is hard work. This study is a testimony to their openness and honesty which the use of pseudonyms belies.

While the surgeons were teaching me that high-quality care is hard work, a number of sociologists were trying to teach me the same lesson about sociological research. This work is better for their support, encouragement, and criticism. Fred Strodtbeck introduced me to the problems with which this dissertation deals, and constantly challenged me to find ways for documenting the reliability and validity of my inferences. Charles Bidwell often saw more clearly than I what I was struggling to say, and was a useful guide through and disposer of needlessly labyrinthine arguments. I owe a singular debt to Barry Schwartz. His insistence that I look beyond the particulars of the field situation to more general social processes improved this work immeasurably. Odin Andersen provided both intellectual and financial assistance through National Center for Health Services Training Grant, HS 00080-08 through 12. Renée C. Fox read and extensively commented on various versions of this manuscript. Her colleagueship and support have been invaluable to me. I cannot do justice to her contribution to this work and to my own growth as a sociologist of medicine in a simple acknowledgment and/or appreciative footnote. Harold Bershady read and gently but firmly critiqued numerous drafts of the manuscript.

Marjorie Waxman, my wife, helped in ways too numerous to

recall. She provided support and encouragement during the very difficult first days of field research; she listened and asked searching questions as I began to develop my analyses; she extended my own thinking by drawing on her own stock of clinical experience; and she insisted that calling an unclear argument "sociological" does little to improve its clarity—her criticisms sent me back to the writing table more times than I like to remember. Were it not for her sense of humor and proportion I would never have finished this work.

A number of friends and associates also provided support, encouragement, and feedback. I am especially thankful to Bruce Atherton, Jarl Dyrud, Margaret Ensminger, Bill and Roseann Gallery, Joel Frader, Jeffrey Hantover, Paul Hirsch, Shepard Kellam, Sue Lelito, Victor Lidz, Jim Lynch, Ann Lyons, Samuel P. Martin III, Peter Meyer, Boyd Slomoff, and Judith Tribbett. The Guttman Foundation generously provided funds for the typing of this manuscript.

Acknowledgments for the Second Edition

In the first edition of *Forgive and Remember,* I noted that fieldwork, like surgery, was a body contact sport. To my great amazement, this was also true for work required to appraise and update the original for this second edition. I am grateful to all the colleagues and friends who did not avoid this contact and whose encouragement and suggestions enriched the final product.

I first presented the material in the epilogue as the eleventh annual Wiese Lecture in Medical Humanities at the Brigham and Women's Hospital, Harvard Medical School. I had an opportunity to present a revised version shortly thereafter as the Ralph W. Caffey Visiting Professor of Surgery, Department of Surgery, University of Missouri Medical School, Kansas City. On both occasions, sharp questions and astute observations from the audience had me rethink points made too hastily.

An invitation to join the project *Humanizing Bioethics: From Abstract Principles to Lived Experience* provided me the opportunity to revisit the fieldwork experience of *Forgive and Remember.* I am glad that Barry Hoffmaster had the vision to propose this working group and that the Social Sciences and Humanities Research Council of Canada funded it. The members of the group—Renee Anspach, Diane Beeson, Michael Burgess, Arthur Caplan, Peter Conrad, Deborah Gordon, Sydney Halpern, Barry Hoffmaster, Bruce Jennings, Sharon Kauffman, Barbara Koenig, Abby Lippman, Margaret Lock, Patricia Marshall, Kate McBurney, and Alison Wylie—provided not only helpful comments on the draft but two years of stimulating conversation on the vexing question of the relationship of social science and bioethics.

Closer to home, students and colleagues provided useful critiques. Elizabeth Armstrong, Jacqueline Hart, Joanna Kempner, and Sita Reddy all had the good sense to recognize that I was serious when I asked for criticism and the good judgment to spot flaws that I had not noticed. Robbie Aronowitz, Harold Bershady, David Grazian, Jerry

Jacobs, Glenn McGee, and Jason Schnittker had suggestions that forced me to revise what I thought was in final form. Robin Leidner rescued me from the passive voice in a very careful editing of yet another not so final as I thought draft. Carla Keirns, drawing on her recent experiences as a medical student as well as her considerable skills as an editor improved the final product. Joel Frader tried, with only limited success, to rescue me from rhetorical excess. Three old friends from graduate school, Jeffrey Hantover, Mark Jacobs, and Jim Lynch provided encouragement, support, and concrete editorial advice at different points in the process.

At home, my daughters Emily and Abigail, by turns, wouldn't let me play when I needed to work and wouldn't let me work when I needed to play. The experience of watching my daughters grow convinced me that I was wrong to omit any discussion of gender in the first edition. Finally, so many years after the original, my wife Marjorie continues to provide support and encouragement, to listen and ask the right clarifying questions, to extend my thinking by drawing upon her own clinical experience, and to reject the notion that imprecise and obscure prose is justified by the label "sociological." Once again her love, support, and sense of proportion made finishing this possible.

A number of friends also provided the support, encouragement, and community that allows the isolation that writing requires. I am especially thankful to Susan Adelman, Carol Avins, Cathy and David Cohen, Margaret and Andy Fichter, Laura and David Henrich, Dan Raff, Jeffrey and Laurel Silber, and Rayman Solomon.

Preface to the Second Edition

A Sociologist Puts
on the Hair Shirt

In the now more than twenty years since the original publication of *Forgive and Remember*, I have never returned to Pacific Hospital. Even so, I have visited enough other academic surgery programs to offer some educated guesses about how Pacific has changed.

For example, if I were to revisit Pacific, I would find new faces—a few of the residents of my original study would now be senior attendings and almost all of the original attendings would have moved on, whether through death, retirement, or natural career mobility. In addition, the current residents would display more diversity than the virtually all-white, male group that was in place when I conducted my research.

I would find new buildings at Pacific. Whatever the fiscal problems of academic health centers—and I am constantly reminded by medical school representatives everywhere that they are baleful and extensive—I am certain that these problems have not impeded construction at Pacific in any noticeable way. I would find new procedures commonplace: fiber-optic devices have expanded the domain of microsurgery, kidneys are not the only organs now regularly transplanted, and the line between radiology that is invasive and therapeutic and surgery has blurred.

I would find that residency has grown more stressful at the same time that the faculty claim that training programs have been scourged of past abusive practices. Talking with residents, I would find that they are skeptical about whether residency has become a kinder, gentler experience. Even if the attending faculty are correct in their Panglossian assessment, residents are taxed with sicker patients who have shorter lengths of stay; there is more work to do in less time. Further, despite an attempt to improve working conditions for residents in other specialties by placing limits on hours, there has been a general resistance to these changes in surgical residencies. Abusive physical demands are still common in surgical residencies. I would find that the haphazard patterns of assessment of resident performance I discussed in the first edition have become standardized. One form this standardization has taken is annual national exams that give surgical residents additional homework after their patient-care duties have been completed. For all that, I would find, as well, that residents are no more certain now than they were then that assessment procedures are fair.

I would also find new departments and services that reflect the bureaucratic sediment of past public problems and reform movements. Pacific, like so many other institutions, now has a bioethics center and an ethics consultation service to help make the difficult decisions that "only an attending" could make when I conducted the original research. The public relations and marketing departments are now a visible presence. I would find new research foci: there is a budding evidence-based medicine and an outcomes research movement, as well as intense activity directed toward mapping the human genome. I would find new diseases: Alzheimer's, AIDS, bacteria-resistant infections (terrifying in surgical patients) such as MRSA (methicillin-resistant staphaureus) and VRE (vancomycin-resistant enteroccus), and bacteria-resistant tuberculosis were not problems when I was in the field at Pacific.

I would find a concern for the financing of care that was not present in the 1970s, expressed through questions about what third-party payers will permit. At the same time, I would find that the formal or informal training that residents receive for managing the health insurance issues that drive both inpatient procedures and outpatient follow-up is scant. This concern for financing has, in turn, been a major force in the expansion of the administrative presence at Pacific. I would find more defensive medicine as well. Since I conducted my fieldwork, there have been three public "malpractice crises" with accompanying concern for the "litigation explosion." I would find that the need of policies to contain costs conflicts with the need of individual practitioners to limit liabilities. The tensions and contradictions created by these two conflicting goals would be easy to observe in conversation, deliberation, decision making, and action on surgical wards. Finally, I would find a new appreciation that medicine is an "error-ridden" activity and a new concern in management policies that reflect the desire to limit these errors and their consequences. The purpose of this new edition is to map what consequences these changes have on the argument of *Forgive and Remember*. I highlight and discuss many of these differences in this edition's epilogue.

II

At the same time, it is not just medicine and its relation to the larger society that has changed since the original publication of *Forgive and Remember*. The conventions of social science scholarship, more generally, and ethnographic reporting, more specifically, have changed as well. Both these changes, and the reasons for them, are too numerous and too complex to catalogue in a prefatory note. Without belaboring that intellectual history here, I think it is fair to say that at the very least, among social scientists who rely on qualitative methods, increased epistemological doubt about the enterprise of ethnography is one consequence of all the changes. Both in anthropology and in sociology, forceful questions have been raised about what it means to observe and to represent the "other." There has been, at times, a paralyzing debate about standpoint, voice, and authorial authority. So much has this been the case that it seems as if the conversation about whether we can and how we should do our work has supplanted the conversation about the work itself. *Forgive and Remember* is, quite evidently, a product of an academic climate untroubled by this debate. It is hard for me to imagine now writing any text so confident in its assertions as the original edition of *Forgive and Remember*. The new fieldwork appendix is, in part, a consequence of all the changes in the conventions of ethnographic reporting, and, in part, a confession of doubts that I had neither the courage nor the cognitive categories to make articulate when the manuscript first appeared.

III

So far, the stately prose of this preface pretends that changes in the social world alone account for the need for a second edition, that there are no defects in the original text that demand extended comment. Would that this were so. But, of course, it is not. In particular, there are two problems with the original text that bother me upon rereading.

First, *Forgive and Remember* provides a trenchant, but not sufficiently appreciative, critique of previous sociological writing on social control in the medical profession. The conventional wisdom of the time was an extended elaboration of Shaw's dictum that "all professions are a conspiracy against the laity." The empirical data for this proposition was found in the relative absence of any action by state disciplinary boards and in observational studies that documented how leniently colleagues treated one another's shortcomings. *Forgive and Remember* tells a different story. This narrative shows how seriously mistakes—especially those understood as normative and quasi-normative—are treated during residency training. I conclude that, above all, residency training is designed as a moral education, the purpose of which is to teach young doctors the standards of practice.

I am not sparing in my criticism of my colleagues who had, to my mind, failed to appreciate this moral dimension of everyday practice. This critique is based on the idea that my colleagues had made a sampling error: they had observed some part of medical practice, made some assumptions about what a robust system of social control would look like, and, failing to find that, concluded social controls were absent. Their failure to find social controls, I argued, stemmed from a lack of appreciation of the inherent uncertainty in the everyday practice of medicine, a definition of error that failed to appreciate the "essentially contested" character of error, and from a reliance on only official sanctions as an index of a serious response to errant performance. Because license suspensions, alternative formal sanctionings, and firings were rare, my colleagues assumed social controls occurred more in the breach than the reality of medical practice. To my mind, my colleagues confused the absent part with the whole.

At the same time, like those colleagues that I take to task, I confuse a part for the whole. First, I observe training in an elite residency. I notice that standards are exacting, that residents are expected to internalize these standards, and that there is the expectation that there will be no erosion of these internalized normative standards over time. While I was certainly aware that Pacific Hospital was in no way representative of all medical practice, and while I indicate that awareness in the occasional parenthetical aside, dependent clause, or hedging endnote appended to the text, I nonetheless make conclusions as if the surgical residency at Pacific were the entire world of medical practice. I pick an argument with colleagues who find social controls almost entirely absent from medical practice. In so doing, I make the same metaphorical and metonymic mistake that I criticize my colleagues for above—I, too, write as if the part is the whole. This creates two different ways in which my conclusions extend further than my data allow.

First, although I am careful to specify that the surgical training program at Pacific Hospital considers itself an elite program dedicated to the production of academic surgeons, and although I acknowledge that there are other surgical training programs with different aspirations for their finished recruits, I write as if the norms at Pacific were shared by all surgical training programs. The possibility that other surgical precincts may operate differently, that they might have different norms, or that they might wink tolerantly at violations that Pacific takes seriously is not something that I sufficiently remind the reader of in the text. This is a significant omission, for with different operative rules, the content of training (that is, above all, moral) will vary, and with different enforcement regimes, the intensity of the lessons in moral education will vary.

Second, I make clear in the text that supervisory authority and norm enforcement coincide with the hierarchy of the resident training program, that social controls are not to be taken for granted without this hierarchy and its accompanying relationships of super- and subordination. I also conclude that greater collegial controls are required so that professional standards can be upheld in everyday settings of clinical care just as they are in professional training. I am vague about how this might happen. However, I fail to consider how norms might shift and change once training is finished. The basic operative norm at Pacific Hospital, the one that was taken most seriously by everyone, the one that was most consistently enforced and least likely to be overlooked, the rule of "no surprises," was directly tied to the hierarchical structure of training. This fact should, at the least, have made me more curious about how social controls looked in settings where hierarchy and subordination were absent. These are, after all, precisely those settings of everyday clinical action in which colleagues had in prior studies found ordinary social controls wanting.

Had I not been so intent on showing that my colleagues who had

found social controls absent were wrong, I might have been able to resolve the contradiction that I saw between the absence of social controls in the world of medical practice as they found it and the presence
of social controls in the world of medical education as I found it. I had
trouble understanding how what I saw so clearly in one setting of care
could be so entirely absent from others. I saw an intense effort to instill
a professional conscience and a sense of what was permissible and
what was not. This effort was indexed by very public disciplinings, the
public scoldings that offended attendings directed at miscreant residents, and by the attendings' practice of "putting on the hair shirt," as
I described it. I saw all of this in the context of the most physically challenging regime that I could imagine. During the period of fieldwork, I
was more sleep deprived and exhausted than I have ever been in my
life. In addition, I saw and experienced all the artifacts of a ceaseless
striving for perfection: an obsession with detail in every aspect of
everyday tasks that was more intense than anything that I had experienced before; a seemingly genuine desire, if not passion, to help others; and real discouragement, disappointment, and even depression
when interventions refused to yield the intended help.

My colleagues who looked at social control in other settings seemed
to find much less passion, dedication, and concern in their clinical settings than I found in mine. I simply concluded that they, with their theoretical and political convictions acting as blinders, failed to see
something that was palpably present to me. I failed to see how my intense immersion in a very unrepresentative segment of the world of
medicine might have acted as blinders for me. I now see that both descriptions may have been accurate. An intense concern for professional norms marks training. An equally strong, structured silence
marks those settings where colleagues are assumed to have learned the
lessons of training. The conclusions and recommendations for change
in *Forgive and Remember* read to me as if I had realized this. The argument preceding those conclusions, regrettably, does not.

This first problem, related as it is to the overgeneralization of one's
findings, the eagerness to display those findings as something wondrous, the desire to show that one has noticed a thing or two that
escaped one's predecessors, and even the overheated prose that accom-
plishes all this, is perhaps excusable as a species of youthful enthusi-

asm—just the sort of thing that happens when one takes oneself too seriously. The second problem is related to the classification system of mistakes that *Forgive and Remember* develops. It strikes me now that the underdevelopment of one of the four types of errors, quasi-normative error, blunts the critical thrust of the analysis. This blunting that I am now about to describe allowed my appreciation of the normative regime of surgical training to shine clearly through the text. However, my aggravation with the arbitrary and capricious operation of attendings' authority when managing quasi-normative error was hidden in the shade of theoretical trees that I had planted but neglected to prune.

In the typology of error that is developed in *Forgive and Remember*, there are four major types of error: technical, judgmental, normative, and quasi-normative. In action, surgeons deploy their understanding of the four types of error to make one truly critical distinction: Is the error blameless or blameworthy? Is the failure of surgical intervention here the result of someone doing what any reasonable person might have done when confronted with that situation as it was understood by all at the time, or is the untoward outcome the result of less than responsible behavior? When errors were classified as technical or judgmental, the residents deemed responsible were seen as blameless. Such mistakes were seen as an inevitable, if unwanted, consequences of training the inexperienced to do cognitively and manually complex labor. However, when errors were classified as normative or quasi-normative, the residents deemed responsible were seen as blameworthy. Such mistakes were not seen as the sort of normal errors necessary for novices to be transformed into adepts. Rather, such mistakes were treated as breaches by a morally accountable agent and as occasion for corrective remedies at the time of the event and more consequential sanctions in the future (especially if further breaches were added to the first).

The very attempt to classify how mistakes and errors were understood has created one trivial type of misunderstanding in the original text. Some have seen technical, judgmental, normative, or quasi-normative errors as exemplars of what philosophers call a "natural" kind. Much in the same way that birders armed with decent binoculars, comfortable shoes, and a good field guide can classify the different aviary species they come across in an afternoon, so could the taxonomist of human behavior armed with *Forgive and Remember* identify the type of errors that are made on surgical units. (In fact, I have even heard of surgical services where residents offer consolation based on their understanding of the text's schema—"Don't worry, it was an understandable technical error," or supportive sympathy—"I once made the same normative error, and I'm still here".) This sort of understanding of Forgive and Remember's classificatory schema displays a misplaced concreteness.

The typology was not intended to suggest that errors had some sort of immutable identity apart from the social setting in which understanding of their occurrence emerged. Errors that were classified one way on one occasion might just as easily be classified another way on another occasion depending upon a staggeringly wide range of contextual factors: who the attending was, who the resident was, how smoothly things were going on the service when the mistake surfaced, how a request for information was managed, what time of year it was when the mistake occurred, how early or late in a rotation the mishap took place, who informed the attending of the problem, and under what circumstances. In any case, my basic intent was to create a taxonomic system that had both clear categories with clear consequences attached to the cognitive pigeonholing (if a, then this; if b, then that) and at the same time allowed for different actors to pigeonhole the same event in different ways based on their understanding of what happened. However flexible the typology was meant to be in theory, it rubbed against an obdurate empirical world in practice. Once an understanding was arrived at, that understanding was fateful for all concerned. The understanding, to wax phenomenological for a moment, "gears into the world" as a somewhat natural, self-evident, and immutable fact. So much is this the case that the failure of a resident to assent to an authoritative understanding of blameworthy error that has a faculty attending championing it, or the attempt by a resident to supply an alternative interpretation for an error, is often taken as evidence of a normative deficit. In all this over-determined certainty nothing is lost, save the sense that things could have been otherwise.

There is a second, more serious misinterpretation to which the schema lends itself; and, sad to say, I am responsible for it. In the text, I note an equivalence of treatment between two types of error, normative and quasi-normative breaches. Although normative breaches involve the violation of universal rules that hold across surgical services and quasi-normative ones involve rules specific to individual attendings and their services, attendings take both violations seriously. In the short run of everyday interaction, these breaches are an occasion for dressing down offending residents, who have to weather the affect storms of their superordinates in open public spaces. In the long run, residents who are seen as guilty of such breaches may find their surgical training at Pacific abruptly foreshortened.

What I do not make as clear in the text as I might is just how many problems in medical training and in the establishment of a culture for patient safety are created by treating normative and quasi-normative breaches in a unitary fashion during surgical residency. Two unfortunate consequences are worth underscoring here. First, the treatment of breaches of universal rules and of specific senior surgeons' individual preferences as if they were the same thing introduces a considerable amount of noise and confusion into the world of the resident who is trying to understand the code of professional conduct that training intends to convey. When breaches that all would agree are serious are treated in the same way as breaches that not all would agree are really breaches at all (or, more precisely, all would agree are only breaches on this service and only because Dr. Whoever says so), then residents have considerable interpretive room when evaluating their own behavior. Serious breaches may be dismissed as "just a matter of Dr. Whoever's craziness" and trivial breaches may be overappreciated with the consequent cost of needless self-laceration and punctured self-esteem. In a field like surgery where much hinges on both the individual's honest assessment of his/her capacities and also on his/her confidence in these skills, these are not trivial costs. The collapsing of normative and quasi-normative breaches in everyday medical practice creates for the resident the problem of separating messages that need be heeded from noise. This dilemma is, of course, not confined to surgical residents and surgical residency. It is part of all clinical training that is dependent on modeling yet leaves it to the individual student to draw their own lessons from the behavior that is being modeled. The collapsing of the distinction between normative and quasi-normative breaches creates interpretive problems for residents as they try to negotiate training; the collapsing of the distinction in the text creates problems for readers as they try to understand the operation of social controls in training. In particular, the failure to make more of the dissonance created by the similarity in treatment of normative and quasi-normative breaches reinforces the illusion of an equitable system that separates the fit from the unfit in a rational fashion. Authority appears benign, aligned with all our better angels. However, the ability of attendings to have their individual idiosyncrasies treated as if they were unalterable, unquestioned universal norms adds an arbitrary and capricious element to the disciplining of residents.

The condensed discussion in the text of this arbitrary element to social control in surgical training impeded a more general sociological discussion of the nature of authority. Generally, professional authority, with its emphasis on specialized theoretic knowledge, is viewed as a highly rational form of authority. What a fuller discussion of the implications of quasi-normative breaches would have made clear is the irreducible irrational element in this and, in fact, all systems of authority. After all, if all authority were fully rational, if it merely commanded us to act in ways that upon reflection we would choose to act because those are the most sensible courses of action, then the compulsive force of authority would rest upon its logic, its superior rationality. However, when authority compels us to act against our own interests, to follow dictates that we find illogical, to submit to definitions of the situation that we find unjust, then authority displays its compulsive force. It is just this element of authority that the discussion of *Forgive and Remember* obscures. The theoretic consequences of this incomplete discussion of authority are made clearer in the new fieldwork appendix.

IV

Since the publication of *Forgive and Remember*, medical errors—or as the policy experts would have it, "preventable adverse events"— have become an issue of significant public attention, debate, and activity. In the fall of 1999, the Institute of Medicine issued a report on error in medicine, *To Err is Human* (Kohn, Corrigan, and Donaldson 2000). The report claims that between 44,000 and 98,000 patients die as the result of "adverse" medical events each year, that over half of these adverse events are preventable, and that these events are the eighth leading cause of death. The report finds that adverse events are not caused by individual negligence but rather by systems of care that pay too little attention to patient safety. The report calls for a multi-pronged attack to end what it calls "the cycle of inaction" with regard to patient safety. Necessary steps that the report calls for include: ending the "name, blame, and shame" culture that inhibits the discussion of adverse events, constructing both voluntary and mandatory reporting systems for adverse events so that lessons from them can be applied widely, and designing a safe system at the point where services are delivered. The goal of the Institute of Medicine's report is to reduce adverse events by half within five years.

This is certainly a laudable goal. However, the argument of *Forgive and Remember* suggests how difficult it may be to achieve. Strictly speaking, *Forgive and Remember* does not focus on what causes error. Rather, it concentrates on how surgeons account for errors once they have occurred. There are three elements of this social accounting system that suggest safety recommendations are easier to formulate than to implement. First, what constitutes an error is, at many levels, an "essentially contested concept." Was this failure the result of error? If so, was the error foreseeable and preventable? And, if so, did the error make a difference to the outcome? *Forgive and Remember* suggests that errors are not events that can be simply counted. Instead, their existence needs to be debated; the discourse over precisely what is and is not an error is necessary to the formation of a sense of professional responsibility. What constitutes an error is an extreme example of "local knowledge." If attempts to reduce error are to be successful, they must grapple with how workers define error, understand its causes, and think it may be remedied. Policy makers also need to appreciate the constraints that workers labor under in order to formulate recommendations that workers will comply with rather than evade.

Next, it is undeniable that a "name, blame, and shame culture" discourages an open discussion of error. There is no doubt much to be gained from reducing this dimension of the culture of physicians, generally, and surgeons, specifically. However, elements of culture do not exist in splendid isolation from one another. In surgery, much depends upon notions of individual responsibility that are inflated and at the same time inimical to patient safety. How is the sense of individual responsibility that is communicated in residency training connected to naming, blaming, and shaming? How do we change one element in a culture without every other dimension of the culture changing with it? Beyond that, as "putting on the hair shirt" shows, attending surgeons do not just blame vulnerable subordinates; they also "name, blame, and shame" themselves. They do this to demonstrate to the community just how seriously they take their responsibilities to patients. That the current culture harms both individual patients and surgeons and, occasionally, degrades safety is without question—the new fieldwork appendix specifies some of those harms more clearly than the original text. This is not a plea to retain "naming, blaming, and shaming." Rather, it is an invitation to think about their relation to the surgeon's sense of professional responsibility, to ask what the limits are to curbing the processes of "naming, blaming, and shaming." It is an invitation as well to appreciate the costs involved in our current practices for instilling a sense of professional responsibility and to think creatively about alternatives. It is an invitation to think about mismatches created by changes in the organization of medical practice and by stasis in the organization of medical training.

Finally, if, as *Forgive and Remember* suggests, the search for errors begins with deaths and complications—begins when the expectation of success is breached—then we have every reason to be skeptical of how practical the recommendation to report "near misses" is. There is much to suggest that physicians have some trouble "seeing" these "near misses." What isn't noticed can't be reported and won't be learned from. *Forgive and Remember* is an extended commentary on how young surgeons learn to "see" error, embedded in that commentary is an explanation of why in a work environment so burdened with production pressures, near misses are so difficult to recognize and attend to. Moreover, those "near misses" that are seen are so obvious as to be trivial. Dangerous "near misses" are, as a rule, only appreciated as harbingers of disaster after disaster has materialized. Until then, they are weak or missed signals. They become clear only with the application of hindsight bias. Once we have the outcome firmly in hand, the causal links are much easier to trace backwards. Working prospectively from only the facts known at the time is more difficult. In general, these remarks on the difficulty of implementing the Institute of Medicine's recommendations are not meant as a counsel of despair. They are intended to urge us to add a dimension to our thinking about patient safety that the report omits, the culture of the workgroup. It is this culture that *Forgive and Remember* details and places at the center of understandings of error, failure, and professional responsibility.

Work Cited

Kohn, Linda T., Corrigan, Janet M., and Davidson, Molla S. eds. 2000. *To Err Is Human: Building A Safer Health System.* Washington, DC: National Academy Press.

one

Introduction

At 6:30 A.M., only a few physicians and staff walk the still-darkened corridors of Pacific Hospital. Within an hour, the hospital will pulse with activity: nurses will wheel medication carts and chart racks down the halls; technicians will draw patients' blood, orderlies will place patients on line for the various diagnostic and therapeutic procedures the hospital provides; vendors will hawk the morning newspaper; and teams of physicians and students will make rounds on their patients. In the predawn, however, there is no hint of the burst of activity to come. A lone houseofficer trudges down the hall. A few nurses from the night shift gather at their station, chat while charting the previous night's activity, and share a last cup of coffee before ending their day at the beginning of everyone else's. Only one small group of physicians is already engaged in the purposive and feverish activity that one associates with the hospital during the day. For them, the day is in full swing. This group of physicians moves from bleary-eyed patient to bleary-eyed patient while jotting down what work must be done that day. Their movements are swift and precise; no energy is wasted in extraneous chatter with patients or each other.

Who are these few physicians? Why are they up so early? They are members of the surgical housestaff of Pacific Hospital. The two or three days a week on which the services they are assigned to operate, these men and women begin rounds at 6:00 A.M. so that they can be scrubbed, capped, gowned, and ready to operate on their first patient at precisely 8:00 A.M. This starting time is important to them for a number of reasons. First, they know if they miss it they will be behind schedule all day. Although the twenty-minute difference between 8:00 A.M. and 8:20 A.M. is not great, it is often the difference between a hurried lunch and a twelve-hour fast. Moreover, this is not a quiet, meditative fast, but one during which the hungry houseofficer must remain standing; assist with or perform operative procedures; pass "ad hoc" quizzes on anatomy and the advisability of various treatment modalities; engage in witty repartee with his superordinate, the attending surgeon; or accept silently his role as butt of his superior's jokes. Second, houseofficers who are not ready on schedule appear to their superordinates as inefficient, lazy, or unreliable. As houseofficers well know, "attendings" do not suffer wasted time—or those who force them to waste it—gladly. A houseofficer's good name rests in part on his ability to keep events running on schedule.

For eighteen months, I was a participant-observer of the surgical training program of Pacific Hospital. Three interrelated problems captured my interest and attracted me to this field setting. First was a question of social control. On precisely what kinds of behavior does a houseofficer's good name rest? What kinds of actions discredit him? How are evaluations of competence constructed by superiors, how are these evaluations shared, and how consequential are they? To use the vocabulary of Everett C. Hughes (1971), I was interested in how a segment of the medical profession exercises its "license" and "mandate."

Second was the question of social support. The superordinate's task is a delicate one. He must control mistakes. Yet at the same time, if he wishes to train competent, independent, and (eventually) autonomous professionals, he must allow his subordinates enough room to make the honest errors of the inexperienced. To allow this requires a certain cold-blooded calculation on the part of the superordinate. On the one hand, he needs to restrain himself from taking charge of situations too quickly lest he damage a subordinate's confidence. On the other hand, he needs to know when to rescue a subordinate—and patient—lest a surgical accident shake the novice's belief in his abilities. So the superordinate has a dual problem: (1) he must control his subordinate's performance and make sure that errors are corrected and not repeated, and (2) he must allow his subordinates room to make errors or they will never learn the judgments and

techniques necessary to perform properly. At all times we should
remember that this give-and-take between ranks is more than a
mere academic exercise; the clinical material for these lessons is
another human being who has placed his life in the surgeon's
hands. Surgical superordinates who are permissive run the risk
of abusing the patient's trust, while those who are restrictive
may retard or destroy the careers of fledgling surgeons. The
forces that lead a superordinate to monitor his subordinates'
behavior more closely or those that lead him to forego close
supervision are therefore not trivial matters. Because the consequences of these different modes of control and support are so
fateful, rationales must be provided for their employment.
Studying the different modes of control and their rationales will
allow us to understand how a group of professionals conceptualizes its privileges and responsibilities.

   Third was the question of sustaining individual commitments,
motivation, and action in the face of failure. How does the
surgeon cope with the knowledge that his clumsiness, forgetful-
ness, or tardiness contributed to another's death and/or suffering? How does the individual surgeon accept this responsibility
and yet not shrink from future action? All groups possess devices
for making failure a normal and accountable feature of everyday
life. Surgeons are no different from the rest of us in this
respect; the difference lies in the consequences of a failure. We
assume that where the possibility of such consequential failure
exists on each and every occasion for action, there will be
powerful, shared devices for coping with these failures. Again,
this is not a trivial matter, for to understand and analyze these
devices is tantamount to analyzing the structure of the profession's conscience: its sense of right and wrong, and its sense of
how large the gray area between them is.

   This report centers on three themes: (1) How a professional
group draws a boundary around itself and determines its own
identity through the selection and rejection of recruits. (2) How
superordinates attempt to control performance and how subordinates accept or avoid such controls in a professional training

program. Of particular importance here is how norms of responsibility to patients and colleagues are articulated and how their violations are sanctioned. (3) How a professional copes with the existential problem of the limits of his skill and of his knowledge. In the course of things a surgeon's best efforts will sometimes fail and he must explain this failure to himself, his colleagues, and the family of his patient. We are interested in how the surgeon achieves accountability to each of these significant audiences and in what situations the surgeon fails to achieve this accountability. Taken together the three issues of membership in a professional group, social control of performance in that group, and shared patterns of explaining, understanding, and neutralizing failure and error are critical not only to our understanding of surgeons but indeed to all of the professions in modern American society.

These are, of course, not new issues; they have been much rehearsed in the sociology of medicine and the sociology of the professions. If these issues are not new, why engage them here? First, I want to recapture and refine the old Durkheimian insight that each occupational group possesses its own morality. I want to specify what for the surgeon is the "complex of ideas and sentiments, [the] ways of seeing and [of] feeling, [the] certain intellectual and moral framework distinctive of the entire group." As an occupational group, surgeons have a collective conscience. I shall make clear what it is, how it is formed, and what functions it serves. I then want to examine how this conscience serves the solidarity of the professional group and at what cost to the larger society. I want to know if any element in this "intellectual and moral framework" defines the essence of a profession in our society. Second, the occupational morality of the surgeon tells us much about how members of a profession interpret, act on, and defend their prerogative of social control. Any programmatic change which intends to make professionals more accountable to clients must of necessity start with a complex phenomenological understanding of what currently passes for accountability and how it is achieved. Field research such as this informs policy by grounding it in a firm understanding of how participants con-

struct their social worlds. It is only from this concrete understanding of the present, practical order that any changes in the
existing interactional politics of social control can be negotiated.

The Field Setting and
Data Collection

The setting for this study of how surgeons detect, categorize, and
sanction error is Pacific Hospital. Pacific Hospital is an elite
medical institution affiliated with a major medical school and
university. In both medicine and surgery, it has a luminous
reputation and a grand tradition. Everywhere one looks, one is
reminded of Pacific's special place in the medical universe.
Portraits of distinguished faculty grace hallways and classrooms.
Lecture rooms and entire wings of the hospital are named after
past greats that Pacific claims as its own. In addition, Pacific
sponsors several endowed lectures a year which are named for its
most eminent embodiments of the clinician-researcher ideal.
These lectures are given by current great names from other
leading medical institutions. This practice underscores symboli-
cally Pacific's great past, its current status, and its hopes for the
future. Its reputation for excellence attracts the top talent to both
Pacific's medical school and residency programs. By and large,
these recruits are considering careers in academic medicine; they
often have strong and well-defined research interests.

   At one time, the splendor of Pacific's medical reputation was
matched by its physical setting in what was once the "gilded"
section of a large urban area. Most of the middle-class inhabi-
tants of the neighborhood have long since moved away and their
elegant mansions have been either leveled or subdivided into
many small apartments. The area that surrounds Pacific is
mostly lower-class black. This population generally uses the
emergency room at Pacific as its primary mode of obtaining
medical care. As a result, the surgical staff of Pacific sees many
patients who are in extreme pain and/or who are the victims of
traumas such as gunshot wounds, beatings, and stabbings. As a
consequence, a good number of the surgical patients at Pacific

meet their surgeons under conditions that are considerably less
orderly than those for typical middle-class patients who are often
referred after some diagnostic tests by their private physicians.
As we shall see later, the nature of a patient's first meeting with
the surgeon is often invoked to explain failure and/or error;
however, for reasons I shall specify, such accounts are never
accepted as legitimate excuses in themselves.

If the splendor of Pacific's neighborhood has faded, that of the
hospital itself has not. Its central shell remains a magnificent
Gothic structure with elaborate stonework, turrets, and gar-
goyles. Attached to the original building are several new wings of
concrete and glass. The original square floor plan of the main
building has with these additions become a bewildering maze of
passageways, tunnels, and crosswalks linking old and new. The
emergency room, the operating rooms, the surgical intensive care
units, X ray, and the patient wards are all located on different
floors in different parts of the hospital. Because of this, simply
carrying out tasks in some logical order is often no mean feat.

Pacific is now approximately a 450-bed structure. Of those
beds, 200 are allocated by the Admitting Office to general
medicine and 193 to surgery. The remainder is for inpatient
psychiatric services. Of the 193 beds allocated to the surgical
services, approximately 120 are reserved for the surgical subspecialties such as neurosurgery, orthopedics, ENT (Ear, Nose,
and Throat), plastics, cardiac and thoracic, and vascular. This
leaves 75 beds or so for all four general surgery services which are
the subject of this report. At Pacific, the general surgery services
perform operations ranging in complexity from removal of
hemorrhoids to esophagojejunostomies [an operation which binds
the esophagus to the upper intestinal tract]. The general surgery
services train housestaff to manage what are considered "normal,
typical," surgical problems, and at the same time the services
perform procedures which would not normally be undertaken
elsewhere because of a patient's compromised condition, the lack
of available support technology, or the presumptive lower level of
competence and confidence of surgeons in other less elite institutions. The general surgery services have two classes of patients:

those referred from colleagues at Pacific or elsewhere because of
the unusually complex nature of their problems, and those who
entered through the emergency room. I did not observe that the
two different types of patients received differential types of care.
Attending surgeons in charge of services stress that they need an
appropriate mix of both patients with complex and routine
problems so that they can keep themselves challenged and at the
same time give their housestaff adequate experience.

During the time of my observations, each of the four general
surgery services performed an average of 24.5 major operations
and 10.2 minor operations per week. The weekly mortality and
morbidity rate, that is, the rate of death and complications, was
5.1. Our task here is not to evaluate whether this rate is high or
low, but rather to explain what this rate means to two groups of
participants, attending surgeons and surgical housestaff. In fact,
one of our first tasks is to see what relationship, if any, exists
between the morbidity and mortality rate—or the official rate of
error—and the surgeon's construction of what an error is and
what its seriousness is. A major focus of this inquiry, then, is the
social processes invoked to construct these rates and the meaning
these rates have for actors in this environment. In this context, it
is interesting to note that each week the Department of Surgery
at Pacific Hospital posts a list of deaths and complications by
service, thereby distributing knowledge of misadventure very
freely within its ranks.

I made observations on two different surgical services: first the
Able and then the Baker (names and identifying characteristics
have been altered). These two different services were chosen by the
logic of the constant comparative method (Glaser and Strauss
1967). The general surgical services at Pacific Hospital varied in
their approach to surgical work along a continuum, the poles of
which were low clinical-high research orientation and high clinical-
low research orientation. Able represented the high research end
of the continuum, Baker the high clinical. The formal division of
labor on each service was identical. At the top of the hierarchy
were attending physicians, all of whom were full-time faculty of
Pacific Medical College whose practices were limited to the pa-

tients on their service. At Pacific all patients were considered the private patients of the attendings whose service they were on: there were no surgical patients who were considered the housestaff's responsibility alone. In a strict legal sense, the attending surgeon was responsible for what happened to patients under his care. It was the attending who decided when to operate and what operation to perform. The attending surgeon was clearly the superordinate on the service. He was the final authority in any disagreements with housestaff; only the attending could give orders binding on every member of the service. Both the Able and the Baker Service had two attendings, each of whom had the final say for his patients. Attendings on a service might disagree with each other about patient care procedures, but each recognized the right of the other to treat his patients as he saw fit and proper.

On each service beneath the two attendings was a chief or senior resident. This resident was responsible for the day-to-day management of patients. He saw to it that the treatment plans of the attending for patients were carried out. The smooth running of the service—making sure that diagnostic tests occur on schedule, that patients do not run into any unexpected troubles, and that all work is done properly—is the chief or senior resident's responsibility. Essentially, he functioned as an attending in the attending's absence; his major task was to anticipate and treat problems before they occurred and to keep the attending informed of these actions. Beneath this level of authority are second- and third-year residents whose precise responsibilities are difficult to state. They must make sure the orders of the chief or senior resident are carried out. They lack responsibility for the entire service but have great responsibility for individual patients. Keeping medications straight, staying up to date on chart work, making certain the patient follows his postoperative regimen (usually walking and expanding the lungs to prevent pneumonia), and maintaining smooth working relations with nurses all seem to be part of this resident's responsibility.

At the bottom of the hierarchy are, in descending order, an intern, a senior medical student, and two or three junior medical students. To use a military analogy, these are the noncommis-

sioned officers of the surgical world. The intern organizes the
students so that the routine but necessary work (scut) of clinical
care is done. Unlike the students, the intern can write medication
orders and admit patients to the hospital. However, his authority
in the hierarchical world of surgery is limited. Surgical interns
often express resentment at how little they are allowed to take
charge of. Senior medical students who may be contemplating
surgical careers receive additional undergraduate exposure to
surgery. For junior students, the surgery rotation is their first
exposure to clinical surgical problems; for many who find surgery
unappealing, it is also their last.

Each service varied at times in how it was staffed; there were
variations in the number of individuals assigned to each service
and in the ranks that were filled. On occasion, there were two
second-year residents; at other times there was only one. On
occasion, there were no senior students. The number of junior
students varied between two and four. Variations in manpower
were unrelated to patient load and were determined by the
scheduling needs of graduate and undergraduate students. Whatever fluctuations existed in staffing, the formal tasks of both
services were identical; preoperative and postoperative care,
operating itself, evaluating referrals from other services, providing
follow-up care to outpatients in the clinic, and supplying emergency room care and continuous coverage for patients of other
services during "on-call" periods. The volume of work and the
proportion of time devoted to each task varied, both among
surgical services and within the same service for different time
periods. Slack periods alternated with periods of frenzied activity. A brief description of the Able and Baker Services, excerpted
from my field notes, follows.

The two attendings for Able Service, Dr. White and Dr. Peters,
run the service from a distance. The two surgeons spend more
time involved in their research activity than they do in direct
clinical care of patients. Dr. White's main research interest is the
problems surrounding organ transplantation. Maintaining the
service allows him to control hospital beds for his kidney transplants. The activity of Able Service is geared to kidney trans-

plants. Periods during which one or more transplants are being performed and/or managed are periods of peak activity; all members of the Able team are animated by a heightened sense of purpose. These periods contrast sharply with those when there are no transplants. Dr. Peters' major interest is research. Both Drs. White and Peters have excellent professional backgrounds and reputations, each having trained with a great name in American surgery. Attending rounds are made by Drs. White and Peters once a week on Saturday morning. They begin at nine in the morning and are over shortly after noon. Neither Dr. White nor Dr. Peters spends a great deal of time instructing residents in surgical techniques; only rarely do they run through a whole operation with subordinates. Chief residents are very active on Able Service; they have a great deal of decision-making power, they get to do a great deal of operating, and they are very much in charge. Residents and interns are not as a rule overly enthusiastic; they are critical of the range of cases that they see and of their actual operative experience. Students, especially those not heavily invested in a possible career in surgery, often relish being assigned to the Able Service since it has the reputation of being a "cakewalk." Dr. White feels that both he and Dr. Peters devote enough of their time and energy to clinical care:

> It all depends on what you mean. I know a lot of patients complain that they don't see us around; they think we're not concerned. What they don't understand is that just because we're not there doesn't mean that we don't know what's going on. I talk to X [current chief resident] every day and so does Peters. I have complete confidence in X. I've helped train him for the last five years. When the year started I really stood over his shoulder; but now I know that if he runs into anything that he can't handle, he'll call me. I live only fifteen minutes away. X can control the bleeding from the worst gunshot wound until I get here. Look, everybody expects Mehta to conduct the orchestra; but they don't expect him to play every instrument himself. Nobody criticizes Mehta when the oboe player hits a wrong note. Well, I lead the service. I don't do everything or watch everything and nobody expects me to. What I do expect is that my residents will keep me fully informed of everything that happens on my service.

The two attendings on the Baker Service, Drs. Arthur and Grant, spend more time involved in direct patient care than do the attendings on the Able Service. Most of Dr. Arthur's research publications are based on his clinical experiences. Dr. Grant does some laboratory work but his current research involves a large clinical series. The Baker Service has the reputation of dealing with the most difficult problems of the four general surgery services. Dr. Arthur specializes in diseases of the colon; Dr. Grant, the biliary tract. Dr. Arthur has a very powerful personality; many of his colleagues and residents think of him as an anachronism, a throwback to the time when surgeons were the prima donnas of the hospital. Dr. Arthur himself is aware of his reputation for theatricality but claims, "It is always well controlled. I use those tricks in very select cases in order to get a very specific response." He states that he learned this theatricality from the renowned surgeon for whom he was a resident. Dr. Grant, on the other hand, is more reserved. In most matters, Dr. Grant defers to Dr. Arthur. Attending rounds are made five days a week on the Baker Service by either Dr. Arthur, Dr. Grant, or both. The attendings use these rounds as their major teaching vehicle; in addition, Dr. Arthur holds a tumor conference once a week to discuss the management of cancer patients; and Dr. Grant meets with students on the service at least once a week to discuss general principles of surgery. Drs. Arthur and Grant are active in teaching surgical techniques to housestaff; they look over their subordinates' shoulders, running through the entire operation with them and giving lessons in basic anatomy to the others assembled in the operating room. Both Drs. Arthur and Grant do a lot of operating themselves. Occasionally, this is a source of tension for the service. Chief residents complain that they do not get enough cases. Residents and interns make the same complaint. By and large, however, housestaff like being assigned to the Baker Service. They state that they get an interesting mix of cases, that they are kept busy, and that both Drs. Arthur and Grant are superb teachers. Some housestaff express a distaste for the service because of Arthur's personality. The Baker Service is busier than the Able Service. It operates more frequently than does Able; and for the period of observation, it had more inpatients and more requests for consultations. Dr. Arthur explains his clinical emphasis as follows:

> Surgery is a body-contact sport, there is no question about it. You can't be a good armchair surgeon. If I want to know if my resident is doing a good job, I have to be in the operating room watching him. I can't tell what kind of a job a colleague has done from just looking at his patient. I may have suspicions but unless I was there and know what kind of situation he was presented with, I can't really say anything. There is no way of telling what kind of surgery was done without watching it. There is no way to teach surgery outside of the operating room that I know of—and I've been in this business a long time.

I made an initial assumption that was incorrect in a way that proved serendipitous. I assumed that, both because of the different leadership styles of the Able and Baker attendings and because of the different emphases of their services, I would have a natural comparison of the ways errors were detected, coded, and redressed in two different social groups, while holding the task constant. However, no interactionally significant differences emerged between the Able and the Baker Services in the handling of errors. What was considered a serious breach on one service was serious on the other. What was a trivial mistake on one service was likewise trivial on the other. More strikingly, the phlegmatic Dr. White and the theatric Dr. Arthur, given comparable situations, tended to respond with the same degree of animation. This alerted me to an underlying uniformity that informed the surgical world view and I began to specify what the elements that accounted for that uniformity were and how when taken together they formed a unique *gestalt*. I began to feel that perhaps Durkheim was more correct than he knew when he suggested that each occupational group had its own unique morality.

During the period of field observation, I made the shared problem that deaths and complications present the work group and the shared and socially patterned ways that emerge for meeting these difficulties the focus of my research. Since these problems do not arise on any scheduled basis, it was necessary for me to follow the schedule of a houseofficer in surgery in order to gather data. This involved following surgeons through their daily activities: I visited patients twice daily on rounds, drank coffee in the doctors' lounge during time-out periods, scrubbed in and assisted on operations when hands were short, stood over bodies as they were pronounced dead, and stayed on call at night and felt the rush of adrenalin that a life-threatening emergency brings.

I systematically varied the ways I interacted with the surgeons. On occasion, I actively questioned them about their actions; on others, I helped wheel the chart rack and medication cart on rounds, was available as a "gofer," and was as much as possible an extra pair of hands; on yet other occasions I observed as quietly as possible. I was by turns a more or less active participant in the scene. I could not correlate any set of roles I assumed with my informants' openness, that is, their willingness to share their thoughts and feelings on the unfolding social activity. The demands of medical work are so great and immediate and the field-worker is such a relatively unimportant figure in the clinical scheme of things that I felt my presence affected the phenomena I was interested in only in insignificant ways, if at all. Whatever the day-to-day or scene-to-scene shifts in the researcher persona, my overarching procedures did not vary. For two to three months, I would be totally immersed in fieldwork; I would go to the hospital six days a week and stay the course of the day. Notes were taken as soon after events as possible, routinely within twenty-four hours. Field notes attempted to record events in as narrative or straightforward fashion as possible. Then, after this intense immersion, I would leave the field for two weeks to a month and perform an "in situ" analysis of my field notes. I developed categories, interpretations, and hypotheses from the field notes and discovered where my data were weak and where my observations needed to be concentrated in the future. I then returned to the field for further observation. In this way I "saturated" my categories and "grounded" my theory (Glaser and Strauss 1967). I left the field only when I was convinced that my observations had reached the point of diminishing marginal utility.

Not all the problems I set for myself could be appropriately answered by data collected by participant observation alone. Among the questions I was interested in was the following: How consequential are negative sanctions to an individual's career path? To get at this question, I had to ask: How do superordinates, attending physicians, construct an evaluation of a houseofficer's competence from observations of the houseofficer's day-to-day task performance? I used two sources of data to supplement my field data: (1) I perused the written evaluations of housestaff by attending surgeons as contained in personnel files (to safeguard individual identities, to preserve confidentiality, all names and dates were removed from the documents before I received them), and (2) I attended the faculty meetings of the Department of Surgery at which the decision to retain or terminate junior housestaff in the training program is made. The process of this decision making has, to my knowledge, never been used in sociological studies of social control in the professions. This is an unfortunate omission since this is one of the few points in a professional career where controls exerted have a formal impact. These decisions serve to allocate medical manpower to different environmental niches in medical practice. The grounds on which these decisions are made reveal much about how effective we may expect the norms of medical culture to be in different environments and hence how effectively we may expect controls to operate.

Once fieldwork was completed, I interviewed those attendings and housestaff with whom I worked most closely. The interviews served two purposes. First, they served as a check on the validity of my data. Many of my interpretations were rephrased as questions for comment. In this way, I could match my assessments against those of actors in the scene; and I could fill in those spots where my observational material was thin. Second, the interviews allowed me to see my observations in a larger context. For example, housestaff were asked to compare their performance on different services. This provided me a fuller picture of their activity and their reaction to it than I could gather from my

field observations. Two different interview schedules were constructed: one for housestaff and one for attendings. These
schedules served as guides rather than formal instruments. All
interviews were kept as conversational as possible. Interviews
lasted between forty-five minutes and one and a half hours. For
attendings the focus of the interview was on how they decided if a
subordinate was good or bad and what they considered to be
unforgivable errors. Of housestaff, I asked what they thought
superordinate's performance expectations were, what they considered to be unforgivable errors, and what they considered the
major difficulties in becoming a surgeon.

        I have collected data on the problem of deviance and social
control among general surgeons in a teaching hospital by a
number of methods: participant observation, perusal of staff
personnel folders, and interviews. I cataloged performance
from several different sources, in addition to my own observations. This triangulated approach to data gathering (see Webb et
al. 1966) gives me confidence in the validity of the inferences
which I have drawn. Often conclusions reached about performance from one data source are confirmed by another.

Theoretic Foundations

This is a field study that asks how surgeons recognize, define, punish, and/or neutralize failure. As a study of social control among
surgeons in an elite academic teaching hospital, this research
adds to our theoretical and empirical understanding of how the
quality of professional work is controlled. To answer these
questions about failure and error I utilize ethnographic methods.
So this study is also an ethnographic account of the ordinary and
extraordinary rites, rituals, and practices which comprise the
everyday life of surgeons. As ethnography this research provides,
I hope, a vivid, resonant description of behavior as it naturally
occurs. With ethnography properly done, ethnographic description has such a sense of verisimilitude, such a sense that "this
must be the way things happen," that the descriptive materials
provide a prima facie case for the validity of theoretic argument,

in this instance a discussion of the nature of social control in the medical profession. At times, unfortunately, the distinctive virtue of ethnography, its phenomenological richness, becomes a vice and one cannot see the theoretic forest for the too-richly described trees. As a result this ethnography, like so many others, runs the risk of being dismissed as "merely description" as if description itself were neither valuable nor necessary. In order to highlight as starkly as possible the way in which doing ethnography is always both a theoretic and a theoretically motivated activity, it is necessary to specify the theoretic and empirical questions that guided this research. After all, it was neither a love of surgeons nor of description that led to this study but rather my sense of what was deeply problematic about deviance, social control, and socialization in the sociology of the professions and the sociology of medicine.

When looking at the literature on deviance and social control in the professions, I have always been struck by the importance of the topic for various perspectives on the professions. Social control is the criterion variable that distinguishes one sociological perspective on the professions from another. Its analytic importance as a variable is matched by its empirical significance because of the policy implications that flow from how one conceptualizes professional behavior. If one follows Freidson, the doctor-patient relationship is an economic transaction in which the physician's primary motivation is to maintain a privileged and protected position for himself in the marketplace. If one follows Parsons, this relationship is one of fiduciary trust in which the physician's primary interest is to safeguard the health of the individual and collectivity. In large part, the policies one advocates at the macrolevel of state and profession are determined by the motivations one thinks operate on the microlevel of doctor and patient. In other words, whether or not the standard *caveat emptor* applies to the doctor-patient relationship is a question of profound sociological and empirical significance; any answer to this question is, of course, dependent on the degree to which the profession takes responsibility for its own social control.

However well or poorly the medical profession has managed

this responsibility, sociologists have analyzed the problem with neither rigor or subtlety. As Janowitz (1976) points out in another context, the term *social control* has had two quite distinct meanings in American sociology. On the one hand, the term is used to refer to an individual or group's capacity to regulate itself on its own initiative. On the other hand, it also refers to the coercive means at a community's disposal to discipline individuals. All of that is to say, social control may be internal or external. It is important to emphasize here that the internal controls are not merely individual or group intrapsychic processes—a family that settles its own disputes, or a work group that disciplines its own members are examples of groups ordered by internal social controls. Furthermore, social control may be formal (judicial process) or informal (an off-the-cuff rebuke). Combining these two dimensions we can derive four analytically distinct modalities of social control.

Informal-internal social controls are the everyday ways that members of a group remind each other of their responsibilities as part of their work routines. For example, as anyone who has had an impulse checked by an innocent question can attest, ordinary conversation exerts a greatly underrated and unappreciated force as a source of control.

All groups possess *formal-internal* means for periodically reviewing their performance. Such institutionalized review varies according to frequency, consequences, formality, and so on. Formal-internal social controls may be blunted by the need and/or desire to sustain pleasant working relations with colleagues. Nevertheless, formal accountability is a regular feature of group life. The case conference in psychiatry, the brown-bag lunch in sociology departments, staff meetings in a bureaucracy —all serve either implicitly or explicitly a social control function.

External controls are those where the individual or group that monitors, judges, and sanctions behavior is neither the individual nor a member of the group whose performance is under scrutiny. The principal who drops in on classrooms, the teacher who gives a surprise quiz, the mother-in-law who visits unannounced in the middle of the day are all using the tactics of *informal-external* control. Such controls are a privilege of rank, which is why school principals are able to employ this method more successfully than mothers-in-law. Random checks are seen by control agents as a particularly effective method of monitoring performance since the performance observed cannot be staged for the occasion. By the same token, those subject to them fear such spot checks since they leave so much to chance.

The official audit is the paradigm of *formal-external* control. Here, there is a regular, ongoing review of performance, standards of acceptable performance are set in advance on the basis of objective criteria, and negative sanctions are attached to failures to meet expectations. Such control mechanisms are highly efficient means for monitoring performance. There appears to be an inverse relationship between moral credibility and formal-external controls: parolees are subject to quite a few, judges virtually none.

In treating social control in the professions, sociologists have not kept even these rather rudimentary dimensions of the term distinct. There is an inability to distinguish internal from external controls and formal from informal ones. Discussing social control in medicine, sociologists have consistently written as if some part stood for the whole. Studies of socialization, deviance, and social control have concentrated on one aspect or another of the paradigm sketched above but they have not seen how the components of it are interrelated nor have they paid close attention to the link between the socialization of physicians and the system of social control.

It is in studies of the socialization of medical students and houseofficers that sociologists have most concentrated on the informal-internal aspects of the work environment. The work of Becker et al. (1961) detailed the processes by which groups of students act in concert to restrict their production as a reaction to what were felt to be the unrealistic and overly burdensome demands of faculty. The Kansas study concentrated rather exclusively on the allocation of student effort and ignored other problems for which students forge collective solutions, such as what is ethical behavior, what is acceptable practice, what makes a colleague trustworthy. Fox (1957a, 1963), in her studies of medical socialization, analyzed how medical students learned to manage their uncertainties and how they learned to strike a balance between detachment and concern. Like Becker, Fox concentrates on the informal-internal cues the student receives from the environment; and, like Becker, Fox neglects to connect this socialization to the area of deviance and social control, especially the individual's latter capacity to monitor, evaluate, and correct his/her own performance. Since internal controls are often learned through informal, if often systematic, ways, and since routines of a work group both establish and enforce the background expectancies against which action is viewed as proper or not, it is clear that a refined theory of social control needs to attend to these phenomena.

The formal-internal mechanisms of social control among physicians have been treated by both Goss (1961) and Freidson and Rhea (1972, 1975). They have observed that such reviews control bureaucratic conditions of work and not the work itself. Direct orders never seem to be given; negative sanctions are rarely, if ever, applied; and advice is offered haltingly, without any attempt to see if it is followed up. Social control mechanisms reinforced by negative sanctions seem not to exist. Such a system either protects the inept, as Goode (1967) suggests, and/or rests on strongly shared norms that presuppose self-corrective action. From the analyses provided we are not in a position to evaluate which of the above is the case, nor are we in a position to assess how these controls are related to those built into everyday activity.

Stelling and Bucher (1972) have described informal-external review. They describe an elaborate set of tactics by subordinates to resist encroachments on their autonomy and a correspondingly elaborate set of countermoves by superordinates to gather information on staff performance. Their discussion of interactional strategies—informative as it is—neglects phenomenological aspects of monitoring: Which acts lead to increased monitoring? What other more enduring negative sanctions go along with increased monitoring? How universal and uniform are the standards that different superordinates apply?

Finally, the absence of formal-external controls—regular audit of practitioner performance or regular recertification—has led sociologists to conclude that if juridical-type controls do not exist then no social controls exist at all. A recent spate of prescriptive treatises in the sociology of medicine (Barber et al. 1973; Crane 1975; Freidson 1975; Gray 1975) all make a similar argument: namely, since the profession itself does not have a well-articulated system of formal controls then regulatory responsibility must be removed from the profession or at least structurally formalized. Whatever the merits of such a strategy—and they are considerable—its rationale rests on the decidedly asociological proposition that the only effective social control is coercive or formal control. Totally dismissed is the notion that individual control or group pressure effectively constrains behavior. It seems to me possible to argue for a more formal system of controls while acknowledging the substantial amount of control that is built into the system through socialization, work routines, and normal relations with colleagues. It is precisely this that a professional dominance perspective fails to do.

There is already a great deal that we know about socialization, deviance, and social control in the medical profession. We know that much role learning takes place informally among peers and that this learning includes aspects of the role that can be evaded as well as those obligations which are sacrosanct. We know that internal regulation concerns more an individual's organization of his/her effort than the quality of that effort. We know that subordinates evade monitoring and superordinates know about and plan for this evasion. We know that colleagues are hesitant about confronting other colleagues with their misdeeds and even more hesitant about applying negative sanctions. We know that an institutionalized system of punishments is so rarely resorted to that for all practical purposes it can hardly be said to exist. We know that some physicians show great dedication, duty, and tirelessness as they pursue their tasks, while others merely go through the motions. We know that those who speak for the profession as a whole are aware that they have within their ranks the slothful, the mendacious, the untrustworthy, and the out-

and-out corrupt; yet corporate remedies for these professional problems are slow to emerge.

There is no debating that the number of coercive or external controls that the medical profession imposes on its members is few. Likewise the number of formal controls that operate is few. Does this mean that controls are entirely absent? If so, how are young physicians socialized to explain away their failures? If not, what are the informal-internal controls? How effective are they? What are their limitations? And how do they articulate with other modalities of control? When the medical profession claims that it controls itself, what does it mean? Is it claiming that its individual members each regulate him/herself so well that any additional controls are unnecessary, or is it claiming that what corporate controls exist are adequate for the task? If the first is the case, how is this remarkable feat achieved; if the second is the case, how do we know? This ethnography explores socialization and social control from the point of view of the surgeon in the teaching hospital. It is an analytical rather than a total ethnography. By this I mean that it is not an attempt to order as fully as possible all dimensions of the surgeon's experience. It is instead a very select crosscut of the surgeon's world in order to answer a very specific empirical question with important theoretical implications, the empirical question being how is social control achieved in this particular environment? I began by taking mortality and morbidity as an indicator of situations in which controls might be appropriate and tried to see from this starting point what physicians regard as an error and what criterion they use to construct error as an objectively given real event, rather than as the arbitrary outcome of any number of independent judgments in an indeterminate sequence of judgments. I am interested in how the physician as a practical theorist establishes "this is what the objects in my world are and this is how they behave," and I am interested in the play of claim and counterclaim by participants in interaction to establish that this is real, this is what happened, this is the way it happened, this is why it happened.

Strange as it seems, what an error is has not been problematic

in previous studies of social control in medicine. Previous studies
have assumed that what counts as an error is a relatively straightforward matter. This is to say that the studies apply, or imply
physicians can and should apply, a standard criterion in identifying error. Error, the object of and cause for social control,
belongs to a class of events with such readily identifiable characteristics that on any occasion its recognition is deemed unproblem-
atic. An event possesses the requisite characteristics and fits the
class or it does not. Moreover, these attributes are specified in
advance of the fact and not determined in a retrospective or ex
post facto fashion. In the literature it is taken for granted that
what counts as an error is easily recognized and agreed on by all
concerned. What is problematic is whether such events will be
punished or go undisciplined. Now, this categorical view of error
displays both a misapprehension of the nature of medical decision making and of the interactional dynamics which surround
social control in a profession.

Medical decision making is a probabilistic enterprise. Presented with a patient with a set of symptoms, the physician makes
a diagnosis and decides on an intervention. Only rarely is it the
case in which the physician can say "this patient has x and we
must do y." Even when it is certain that a patient has x, this does
not dictate what should be done since the treatment of choice will
vary according to the severity of x, the patient's age, the
physician's skill, and the technology available at any given
hospital. Moreover, there are some disorders for which there is
significant disagreement among equally learned colleagues over
what the treatment of choice should be. Finally it is not always
clear that a patient has x since there are any number of disorders
with similar symptoms. Whatever may be the nature and depth of
his uncertainty, the physician is usually forced by the patient's
condition to act before that uncertainty is resolved. In this
situation, the physician's action is dictated by what he knows at
the time. I am not denying that there are diagnostic errors made
during the initial contact of physician and patient and that some
of these are sustained until the patient's death. What I am saying
is that not all diagnoses and treatments that later experience

proves wrong are mistakes; some are actions that any reasonable physician would have made under the circumstances. It is plainly not possible to understand how the social controls in the medical profession operate unless one understands how physicians draw the line between what was a reasonable treatment option that subsequent events proved wrong and a course of action that was indefensible given the facts at hand, an error.

Because we as medical sociologists have not understood the difference between these two types of events, because we have given error an unequivocal ontological status, we have missed a step in analyzing the negotiated order of social control. The characteristic slowness of, the hesitation surrounding, and the lenience of professional control in medicine has been well documented; but how physicians view such practices and why they allow them has not. What counts as an error—that set of background understandings, norms, and values that are invoked to categorize clinical events as blameworthy error or blameless misfortune—has not been explored. We have been quite glib in describing how errors are treated, but we have neglected to explain what errors are. The sociologist's understanding of error diverges in a fundamental way from the physician's. For the physician, error is what W. J. Gallie (Lukes 1977) calls an "essentially contested" concept. By this term, Gallie means to convey the inevitable indeterminateness of certain socially constructed categories, such as beautiful or merciful. There are grounds for debating the appropriateness of these concepts on each and every occasion of their use. For the physician, error is just such an essentially contested concept. In this report, I first ask how error is defined, by whom, and under what circumstances; and then I ask how it is managed. Because of my extensive and intensive field experience, I am able to do this from the point of view of others—the surgeon who has made an error, the surgeon who has discovered one made by a colleague, and the surgeon who is responsible for seeing that such a breach is both corrected and not repeated. I do not take the point of view of the patient since the occurrence of error is usually concealed from him and since he does not enter the interactions which surround social control. However lamentable the fact, the patient is an exogenous variable falling outside the system of social control.

While starting with the question of what is error rather than how it is managed does not appear a momentous matter, it promises to advance our understanding of the professions, both as occupations with the special privileges and burdens of rank, as collectivities with rituals for celebration and for mourning, and as fraternities with means to close ranks for self-protection and preservation. By asking what an error for a surgeon is in particular and for a physician in general, I avoid prejudging the adequacy of the modes of social control, but concentrate instead on how this activity is accomplished. Moreover, raising the question in this fashion allows me to explore some recurrent issues on the nature of professions in our society. First, there is a general consensus among sociologists that professions are distinct from other occupational groups by their claims of both a body of theoretic knowledge on which practice rests and a special code of conduct which governs relations among colleagues, clients, and the general public. It follows then that there are two possible sources of deviance. On the one hand, there is the body of theoretic knowledge. Mistakes are made in either judgment or the application of techniques. On the other hand, there is the code of conduct on which professional practice rests. Mistakes are made in the interpretation of norms, that is, the moral standards of the community. Are mistakes, whatever their source, treated the same or is one type of mistake treated more seriously than the other? Do those two types of events occur with equal frequency?

Second, although many sociologists have indicated in a very general way the range of responses to error among physicians, they have failed to link performances to sanctions—that is, they have engaged the issue of social control only after physicians have made the diagnosis of colleague error. I ask by what criteria do surgeons make this diagnosis and what treatments do they view as appropriate given such a diagnosis. My goal is to make clear the fit between the type of error and the type of response it provokes in a community of professionals.

Third, we do not know what types of "recovery work" physicians are forced to do to make failure excusable nor do we know what kinds of failure are considered unforgivable. Given the diffuse uncertainty that surrounds medical diagnosis and decision making, errors attributable to the body of theoretic knowledge may be more easily neutralized than those attributable to the code of conduct since presumably there is much less uncertainty here. Even so, it may be the case that each type of error has its own specific mode of recovery work unique to it. Certainly there are mistakes that physicians make from which patients never recover. Are there mistakes which physicians make from which they themselves cannot recover, which are fatal to their careers and their standing in their colleague community? What are these?

Fourth, we do not understand the effects of available punishments and controls on career paths. Sociologists have long been interested in career paths; in high-status, highly competitive fields such as medicine and surgery, we often make the assumption that one earns one's position. Should we not also entertain the idea that some career niches are a form of exile and punishment, whatever the material rewards, and that some physicians inhabit these niches as a result of professional misdeeds? I explore how social controls sort physicians into different work and career spaces. I examine how consequential the everyday evaluation of performance is for the physician's career. Do negative sanctions have very short-lived effects or do their effects live on and affect a physician's entire career?

Fifth, we do not know how recruits to a profession learn what the standards of performance are, learn the difference between forgivable and unforgivable failure, and learn for themselves how to interpret professional license and mandate. By observing the social control of error among surgical housestaff I can explicate a neglected dimension of medical socialization; namely, how a physician forms his sense of what is professionally right and wrong. During training one learns how to discriminate humanely avoidable from absolutely inevitable failure; how in the case of avoidable failure to distinguish between innocent and blameworthy mistakes; and how, in the case of blameworthy mistakes, to do penance for misdeeds. This is to say, that through socialization, a professional superego develops, models of acceptable behavior are formed, and models of atoning for unacceptable behavior are learned. We assume that these models exert a continuing influence throughout an individual's career—their strength being contingent on their reinforcement in the workplace. However, we know little of their continuing influence because we know so little about the formation of the norms of clinical practice.

In short, our lack of understanding of how physicians detect, categorize, and punish error is fatal to our understanding of social control in the medical profession. Because of this, we do not know how to interpret a profession's claim to be self-regulating. We have no idea of the interplay of event, claim, and counterclaim from which professional deviance and social control is constructed. In this report, I shall look at the patterns of behavior that determine whether an event is labeled an error or not; examine the factors that determine the gravity of an error, independent of its effect on a patient; analyze how individual actors understand the rules for labeling error; and see how these rules help form a hierarchical, but very limited authority system which has very concrete implications for the quality of care we all receive.

Why Surgeons?

A fair question at this point is, Why study one group of surgeons at one elite teaching hospital in order to determine how error is detected, categorized, and punished among physicians? Has sociology as a discipline not developed techniques that lead to generalizations that are valid for a larger population and that lend themselves to easier replication? To argue for some approach to this problem other than an ethnographic one misses much of what I have had to say thus far about the nature of medical decision making and errors. My choice of method, site, and subject was guided first and foremost by theoretic concerns. I have argued that error is an "essentially contested" concept. By this I mean that the grounds for fixing the label "error" to any action are always arguable. In two similar cases with identical outcomes one person may be considered guilty of an error while the other is blameless. Our task in this report is to account for this difference. We need to see under what circumstances, by what criteria, with what consequences, for which audiences an act is or is not considered an error. There is quite simply no other way to do this other than by observing physicians as they account for cases where outcomes fall short of expectations. In this way alone can we determine on what grounds the label "error" is contested and what grounds are essential to establish the label.

Even so, the logic that dictates a field study, that is, the vague, relative, and emergent qualities of the category "error," does not compel us to look at surgeons. We could just as well observe psychiatrists (a favorite pursuit of sociologists) or cardiologists or neurologists or dermatologists. We could look at two or three specialties and compare the way errors are treated within them. However, there are qualities peculiar to the practice of surgery that make surgeons the most appropriate object of our study. In fact, these same qualities allow surgeons to be singled out by critics of health care as it is currently organized as prime abusers of the public trust. Impressive statistics on unnecessary surgery, highly publicized malpractice settlements, sensational media accounts of criminal incompetence and neglect have all combined to make the surgeon a dramatic symbol of what is wrong with the profession of medicine. There is some poetic justice in this. After all, the surgeon who performs under a spotlight in an operating theater was for years the prima donna in the hospital and the object of public adulation. Parsons (1951) has even suggested that surgeons as instrumentally active, pragmatically oriented individuals who take decisive action to save human life display value patterns and behaviors that are emblematic of the "hero" in American society. Worthy of note in this respect are the many popular culture presentations of physicians that feature surgeons such as Ben Casey, Joe Gannon, or the M.A.S.H. medics. We are all familiar with the de rigeur nature of the decisive operation in hospital drama. The features of surgery that make surgeons

"heroes" from one point of view at one point in time and that
make them symbols of corruption, mendacity, and greed from
another point of view at another time are the very features that
make surgeons so well suited to serve as subjects of this report.
These features are the precise and definitive nature of surgical
intervention—its visibility, the expectation of success that surrounds this intervention, and the relatively short time frame in
which outcomes are known. All of these make surgeons more
accountable than their colleagues in other specialties.

Surgical interventions are very precise and definitive. The
surgeon cuts into the body and removes or rearranges various
body parts in order to cure or palliate disease. For patients,
surgery is intrusive and radical therapy. The specific nature of
surgical treatment links the action of the physician and the
response of the patient more intimately than in other areas of
medicine. In many branches of internal medicine the physician's
interventions are relatively nonspecific. This fact allows internists
to attribute failure to the inevitable pathophysiology of the
disease process rather than to the nature of treatment itself. In
psychotherapy, where goals are often diffuse and treatment is
neither precise nor definitive, Light (1972) has demonstrated that
in cases of failure the actions of therapist and the response of the
patient are not seen as linked. Light reports that the normative
belief that the patient alone is responsible for his actions and his
life is routinely invoked following suicide, when the imputation of
therapist error is strongest. Precise, definitive interventions with
very specific expectations make failure to achieve objectives a
more salient issue than in areas where interventions are nonspecific and expectations diffuse. Of all physicians, the surgeon's
interventions are most visible and his therapeutic expectations are
most specific. These features intimately link the surgeon's action
to the patient's condition.

So clearly are the surgeon's actions connected to the patient's
condition that the only warrant for surgery—the only acceptable
reason to subject a patient to the risk and trauma of surgery—is
the expectation that the operation will cure or palliate the
patient's condition. The expectation of success is the background

understanding which legitimates surgical action. Such an expectation does not govern action to the same degree in other
specialties. To understand this point, let us compare two examples. If a surgeon operates on an eighty-three-year-old patient
with gallbladder problems and the patient dies, then the surgeon
cannot very well make the claim that the patient died of old age.
He must first explain how and why the patient received a scar on
his abdomen. Now, an internist medically managing the same
gallbladder problem with the same result can legitimately claim
that the patient died of old age. Deaths and complications
present different questions to different specialists. When the
patient of an internist dies, the natural question his colleagues
ask is, "What happened?" When the patient of a surgeon dies his
colleagues ask, "What did you do?" By the nature of his craft
and his beliefs about it, the surgeon is more accountable than
other physicians and he also has much more to account for. Of
course, this is not all to say that every time a surgical patient dies
the surgeon is at fault, only that it is much harder for him to
claim that he had no hand in it than it is for other colleagues.

The expectation of success which is the only warrant for
surgery compels the surgeon to be more sensitive than his
colleague to the implicit indictment of his skill and/or judgment
signified by therapeutic failure. But to say that there is an
expectation of success is to recognize the possibility of failure. In
a very real way every time a surgeon operates, he is making book
on himself. Besides the enormous amount of theoretic and
technical expertise that is his cognitive capital, the surgeon
carries in his head an odds-book for each procedure he performs; he knows the mortality and morbidity attached to each
procedure; and he is able to revise these odds up or down on the
basis of each patient's age and physical condition. The risk taking implicit in surgical action makes surgical failure a double-
edged sword: one may avoid charges of technical incompetence
only to be accused of reckless judgment. Because of the nature of
the surgeon's risk taking on the patient's behalf, a comprehensive
look at surgeons lays bare many social and ethical dilemmas
which modern medicine faces. Among these are How is the

Hippocratic injunction, "First, do no harm" to be interpreted? What is acceptable risk? How are scarce healing resources allocated? What constitutes informed consent? What is the trade-off between technical virtuosity and compassionate healing?

Because of the visibility of their actions and the expectations that surround them, each death and complication raises the question of error and responsibility for surgeons in a very direct way. By observing the shared and socially patterned ways that surgeons treat deaths and complications, we shall see how surgeons discover and label failure, how they attempt to avoid the implicit indictment of their skills attendant upon failure, and how they punish whoever are deemed culpable parties. However, I am not just observing any surgeons, but surgeons in an elite, academic enviroment. It is reasonable to ask, How is this practice setting distinct from more modal ones? First, increased account-ability is generic to surgery, but it is possible that mechanisms for actually achieving this accountability are not equally present in all practice settings. I assume—and my informants report—that both formal and informal mechanisms for achieving account-ability are more available in elite than in nonelite settings. To be elite means to assume a stance of "first among equals." In elite settings the practice of surgery focuses on difficult surgical cases that represent what is presumptively "the cutting edge" of the field; the major concern is for the elegance of surgery—its artful dimensions—uncontaminated by such mundane matters as fees and their collection, social exchanges to generate referrals, and so on. Where preeminenece is unquestioned, there may be a greater willingness to explore the reasons for failure. This is all the more so in an academic environment which encourages technical talk about a case in a theoretic manner so that unfortunate results may be detached from those that caused them.

There is a second reason for assuming that mechanisms of social control are more prevalent in our setting. Apart from the consequences of its elite reputation, Pacific is an academic institution. Ranks of superordinates and subordinates are quite distinct; the hierarchy is extremely visible and is known to all. Since a part of any socialization process is both positive and negative reinforcement, we would expect the informal-internal processes of control to occur more commonly in teaching institutions. We would expect this quite apart from the fact that superordinates can and do limit subordinates more easily than they do colleagues. So our site, we assume, differs from more modal settings in that at the very least the very processes that we were most interested in would be more present than in other settings. I assume that the general patterns I found hold in all settings. For example, I found that what I call technical errors are always subordinated to what I call normative errors. I assume that this is true for all settings. What I do not know is how universal versus how situated professional norms are; so as a consequence, I cannot describe whether the norms of Pacific's surgeons are shared only by other members of the academic elite or by all surgeons. This is certainly an important issue, but it does not alter the general argument that I make about the relation of individual to corporate controls in the profession nor does it alter the arguments I make about how the legitimacy of quasi-normative or idiosyncratic standards undermine the control process. My site selection limits the universe to which I can generalize, but at the same time it provides a setting in which controls are both salient and displayed in their most primitive form. It allows us to see most clearly what surgeons consider an error, why they use this definition, and how they enforce it.

Conclusion and Overview

I have argued that discussions of social control in medicine and the professions are flawed because they take what an error is for granted. Such studies ignore the phenomenological nature of error as a category of social life and the probabilistic nature of medical decision making. I have attempted to remedy this defect through a field study of surgeons at Pacific Hospital, an elite urban institution. I spent my time on two different services; first, the Able—a high research–low clinical orientation unit; and then, the Baker—a high clinical–low research orientation unit. During my fieldwork, I made failure in the everyday life of the physician and the shared and socially patterned ways that emerge for dealing with it my focal concern. I explain how failure is recognized, managed, controlled, and denied. Since by virtue of their task structure and norms of accountability failure is such a salient question for surgeons, I made them the subjects of my inquiry.

In the next chapter, I will explore the various interpretations of failure that surgeons routinely employ. Four definitions categorize failure—technical error, judgmental error, normative error, and quasi-normative error. Normative and quasi-normative errors alone challenge a surgeon's claim of competence. Chapter 2 shows how these definitions of failure are negotiated and how these labels for failure are related to the division of labor. We are concerned here with the articulations of the division of labor and responsibility.

I turn, in chapter 3, to the various everyday methods superordinates employ to keep error at a minimum. I shall show how these control tactics involve encroaching on the autonomy of subordinates; and I shall describe how subordinates resent and resist this encroachment. In so doing, I shall explore the tension between the two competing systems of legitimation in the medical world: rule by clinical experience and rule from scientific evidence. Second, I examine the questioning process that superordinates use to assign errors to one category or another. Third, I shall analyze the "horror story" as a key element in the oral culture of the medical world and show how it functions as a social control mechanism.

Chapter 4 explores formal peer review in surgery. In this chapter, I show how surgeons account for the "normal troubles" of their craft. I develop a paradigm that allows us to typify these normal troubles and to show the tactics of interpretation surgeons use as a routine part of the "recovery work" for failure. I then analyze a peculiar ritual which occurs in formal peer review sessions: "putting on the hair shirt." Here, superordinates admit error and humble themselves before an audience of colleagues and subordinates. I shall explain the nature of these ritualized admissions of fallibility.

In chapter 5, I explore the impact of failure on a subordinate's career path. I shall show what breaches the surgical profession considers tolerable, and what breaches are unforgivable. I shall explore how the day-to-day performance of subordinates is evaluated and how the judgment "this is a promising surgeon" is constructed. In this analysis we can see the operation of license and mandate collapsed into a single act: the promotion and dismissal of recruits.

Chapter 6 concludes the study by showing how professional self-control operates. I show how professional deviance is identified. I demonstrate how controls operate. I assess one consequence of this definition of the situation: the hypertrophy of individual controls and the atrophy of corporate control. I also present a methodological appendix which describes how I collected and coded my data and how I made myself a part of the surgeon's routine environment.

two

Error, Rank, and
Responsibility

When deaths and complications disturb the surgical expectation of success, those involved are compelled to find good reasons to account for failure.[1] A grammar of motives is manipulated to find an acceptable answer to the question, What went wrong?[2] Moreover, deaths and complications are only one way in which surgical action is disrupted. Nurses and housestaff quarrel; diagnostic procedures do not occur as scheduled; patients fail to follow surgical regimens; and worried families disturb what are, for the physician, the most prosaic of procedures with questions, requests for more information, and demands for reassurance. All of these activities—in addition to the failure of surgical intervention itself—lead attending surgeons to question a houseofficer's competence. None of these events is a failure in and of itself, but all such events carry failure's frightening imputations. These events are occasions for negotiating whether a failure did in fact occur, whether that failure is a result of individual error, and whether or not that error is excusable.

The failure to sustain orderly surgical activity[3] varies in intensity as a threat to a subordinate's competence, depending on how rudely expectations are breached, how frequently an individual breaches expectations, and how easily, if at all, the action may be reversed. This chapter explores the meanings that are negotiated in the wake of breached expectations, relates these meanings to the division of labor, and explores how these meanings are fateful for those involved. The explanation of failure has far-reaching ramifications since it morally typifies the person who is considered responsible. My concern here is with only the informal working understandings of superiors and subordinates that sustain continued action in the face of failure. Later I will discuss formal negotiations, as they occur in peer review, and formal evaluations of performance, as they occur among attending surgeons when tracking housestaff into different career paths.

A surgeon's attempts to explain preventable failure may be divided into four categories: (1) technical error, (2) judgmental error, (3) normative error, and (4) quasi-normative error. Although other interpretations of failure exist, only these four categories deal directly with the issue of physician competence and the social control of performance. Other labels are an attempt to locate responsibility in an area outside the surgeon's control, and are thus often of questionable legitimacy because of the highly developed ethic of individual responsibility among surgeons.

Technical Errors

When a surgeon makes a technical error, he is performing his role conscientiously but his skills fall short of what the task requires. Technical errors are expected to happen to everyone, but rarely. They are expected to happen to everyone because surgeons understand that theirs is at best an imperfectly applied science. At times, interventions fail because techniques have been less than perfectly performed. Certain failures of technique are expected as a routine and calculable part of the work environment: they are built into training. Knots tied by the unpracticed may leave dead space for infection or may split; probes and scopes in the hands of the inexperienced may explore more of the body than desired:

> There are always complications from unfamiliar techniques. A resident may get a pneumothorax [air or gas introduced into the pleural cavity] when he taps a chest, or he may get a hematoma [a large bruise] after a procedure. If these things didn't happen to him, he wouldn't need us; he'd already be a professor of surgery. These things still happen to me but not nearly so often. They are the reason we have a training program, so housestaff can learn to do procedures without incident (Attending).[4]

Further, attending surgeons claim that they can forgive even the most serious lapses in technique, the grossest of mistakes:

Look, suppose when a resident opens the abdomen he nicks
the aorta—now that's dumb, stupid, anything you want to call
absolute incompetence; I mean, the only way to do that is to
really dig in with the knife. It's plain dumb, but it's not
unforgivable. It's a mistake and everybody makes mistakes
one way or another. Our job is to minimize these mistakes
and give people the kind of training that makes them rare
(Attending).

Certain failures are then interpreted as technical in nature. They
are seen by attendings as an occasion for passing on to apprentice
surgeons the "tricks of the trade." Such failures highlight a
training definition of the situation. In cases of technical error, the
role-relation of attending and houseofficer is that of teacher and
student.

For an error to be defined as technical, two conditions must be
met. First the error has to be speedily noticed, reported, and
treated. Such a chain of events serves as a signal of the subordinate's good intentions at the same time that it allows treatment of
the problem before it becomes unmanageable. The same objective
condition reported immediately on one occasion and later on
another will meet with a different response from attendings.
Given the inevitability of problems, their speedy report underscores a houseofficer's conscientiousness and his concern for the
patient; it pays tribute to the norms of clinical responsibility at
the same time that events themselves mock these norms. As we
shall see, a slow discovery of a technical error leads attendings to
suspect that more than a technical failure was involved; they
begin to think a moral lapse may have been involved as well.
Moreover, quick reporting of error maximizes the possibility of
routine remedies and thus minimizes for all the cost of failure.

We left Julio Jimenez's room after rounds. Mark, the chief
resident, shook his head and spoke: "I had bad dreams about
Julio all night. He's got this horrible infection going on in his
belly; and I can't figure out what's causing it. This infection is
clearly the result of some technical error. It could have been
caused by any of a multitude of factors, really. But it's a
technical error, no doubt about it. Fortunately, for us and for

him, Carl [the intern] noticed it right away or else he'd be
awfully sick and we'd have a real mess on our hands"
(Able Service).

It is nevertheless important to remember that the costs of
technical failure never shrink to zero, and it is the patient who
always pays. The patient pays financially in increased hospital
costs and pays personally in the discomfort of a complication. For
subordinates, quick report of failure is one of the primary means
of establishing that the error is not representative of its maker,
that it signals only a momentary lapse, and that it occurred
merely because of its maker's inexperience.

A second condition must be met for failure to be defined as
technical; mistakes must not be frequently made by the same
person. When an individual makes mistakes frequently, he cannot legitimately claim that a momentary lapse occurred. Moreover, attendings would not accept such a claim because frequent
failure makes them doubt not only a subordinate's efforts but also
his intentions:

> When a person makes the same mistake over again, you know
> you're not getting through. For example, if a person comes
> into the operating room and he's tying knots improperly, then
> you tell him, "You practice tying knots on your bedpost and
> not my patient." And if the next time you're in the operating
> room he's doing the same thing, you can see that he's not
> making progress. And if he's not applying himself in one
> area, he's probably not applying himself in others (Attending).

In fact, when an error occurs, attendings ask themselves how
often this housestaff member has been involved in this sort of
thing:

> When you see residents make a mistake, you ask yourself:
> "Are they repeating the same mistake?" It's a matter of
> memory. To be frank, it's holding a grudge. I'm sure you've
> heard us say: "Forgive and remember." When you see some-
> thing, you ask yourself: "Has that happened before? Is it a
> pattern?" (Attending).

For their part, housestaff are worried not so much about making a mistake as failing to learn from those mistakes that they do make. They report, almost universally, the same feelings: at the beginning of their training they are terribly afraid that they will make errors that will have disastrous consequences for patients. Then they learn that they and all those around them make mistakes and that generally the consequences of such mistakes can be managed. Finally, they fear repeating the same mistakes and not learning from their experience. However, all report that their errors are etched indelibly in their memory:

> Of course I worry about making a mistake and it really being disastrous for a patient. But really the crime is not making a mistake; everybody is going to make mistakes. The crime is not learning from your errors. What is really inexcusable is making the same mistake twice. For example, once I can remember sending home a young girl who came into the emergency room at four in the morning and who had abdominal pains and couldn't urinate. I was lucky somebody read over what I had done the next day and said: "Good God, get her back right away—she has appendicitis." So they brought her back and operated that afternoon and she did have appendicitis. That was a case of me not knowing enough and making the wrong decision, but nothing like that will happen again. I learned from it (Intern).

> Mistakes bother you less and less as you go on. I was really sensitive when I started. Fear of doing something wrong and being yelled at was a real motivating factor for me at first. I combatted the fear by working hard and paying a lot of attention to detail. During training you find out mistakes are not such a bad thing and that everybody makes them. But my first year I was extremely afraid. I became less afraid as I went along, but I also made fewer mistakes because I had more experience (Chief Resident).

This knowledge—that a mistake once made should never be made again—is a commonsense understanding that allows both housestaff and attendings to face the unpleasant fact that, because they carried out a task less than competently, another individual was caused to suffer. Technical errors and their lessons are even transformed on occasion into positive experiences. Benefits of the error are believed to outweigh the costs. One individual suffers, but legions of patients yet unseen have the lesson gleaned from this error passed on to them. Moreover, attendings need a certain number of errors in order to teach housestaff how to avoid common problems or how to meet them when they arise. Housestaff need exposure to a wide range of problems so that when training is completed, they are prepared to meet any of the contingencies which disrupt surgical action.

Be that as it may, neither attendings nor housestaff are sanguine in the face of technical error; and every effort is made to keep the number of technical errors small. While the acceptance of technical error is easy as a long-run and abstract proposition, concrete instances are most unwelcome. Work is organized on a surgical service in order to suppress the absolute number of technical errors. Two factors are most noteworthy. First, there is the technical division of labor which is arranged so that subordinates do not advance to complex tasks until they have demonstrated their competence at simpler ones. Before doing nonoperative procedures on their own for the first time, housestaff are shown how by more experienced service members and they are routinely monitored the first time they perform a task. Operations are performed by housestaff under the watchful eyes of attendings or more experienced residents who give advice during the procedure. So much is this supervision expected that when it does not occur, subordinates feel abandoned by superordinates:

> Paul, a second-year resident, was to perform his first colostomy [opening and externalizing a segment of the colon] on Mr. Herman, a patient with cancer of the rectum. Dr. Peters, Mr. Herman's attending, entered the room before the procedure began and asked Paul if he had ever done one of these before. Paul said he hadn't. Peters told him it would be no problem, that they would whip right through it. Peters then took a marking pencil and drew a line on Herman's abdomen indicating how he'd like the body opened. Peters then turned to Paul and said, "Scrub and begin. I have one or

two things to take care of, but I'll be back to help you." Paul
scrubbed, prepared and draped the body, and began the
operation. Peters never returned. Paul began to grumble as he
did the procedure. A few times he asked the scrub nurse for
instructions: What type of suture was normally used? How big
an incision should he make to bring the colostomy out? How
much bowel should he exteriorize? and so on. As soon as the
procedure was finished, he sought out Able's chief resident,
Mark, and complained: "Listen, if I had known Peters wasn't
coming back, I would never have done that alone. I didn't
know what I was doing." Mark did what he could to calm
Paul, who was very upset. Mark kept pointing out how well
the operation had gone. Paul remained unconvinced
(Able Service).

Such breaches are, however, rare; and it is these exceptions and
the strong feelings that they mobilize that allow us to infer how
much a tightly controlled, well-supervised division of labor is the
norm.

A more common problem is the reverse situation: beginning
housestaff feel that the training process moves too slowly and that
they are not getting enough experience or enough opportunity to
exercise their judgment:

In the dinner line this evening, Brian, an intern, was
complaining to Josh, a second-year resident, about doing
a breast biopsy with Ernest, Baker's chief resident. Brian
said, "I lost my biopsy to Ernest today." Josh asked, "What
do you mean? Didn't he let you do it?" Brian answered,
"Yeah, he let me do it. But he's real intrusive to work with.
He couldn't keep his hands out of my operative field. If that
ever happens again, I'll refuse to scrub with him again"
(Baker Service).

The threat is idle, but the complaint is real. We should be alert to
the fact that when this incident occurred Brian had been an
intern only a month, yet he already felt the control of work
confining. Another event a few days later further illustrates the
point:

After rounds, Ernest broke off from the rest of the Baker
Service and went to the outpatient department to do a biopsy.
After he left, a junior student asked where he had gone. Brian
answered, "To do a junior student case." He then turned to
me and went on without prompting, "Ernest takes a lot of
cases that a chief resident has no business touching. Cases
that Josh and I should be doing. It's really frustrating—he
just grabs up everything." I asked Brian why Ernest would do
this. He responded, "It's because Arthur and Grant do things
that you just don't expect attendings to touch. So Ernest
never feels he has enough to do. So he takes cases from Josh
and then Josh takes cases from me. It's all very frustrating"
(Baker Service).

The argot of a surgery service associates operative problems
with rank: a "junior student case" is a simple procedure, one for
the most untrained; and an "attending case" is the most difficult
of procedures. To accuse the chief resident of doing junior student cases is therefore to make a serious complaint about the
division of labor and responsibility. Nevertheless, what is at issue
here is not whether the two attendings hogged cases; on the same
service at the end of the previous training year, there were no
complaints about the division of labor. Control of work and
supervision is most intense during the early stages of the training
year and relaxes as training proceeds and subordinates gain exposure to and experience with new techniques. We should not be
surprised that the graduates of elite medical schools find a rigid
division of labor frustrating, but neither should we overlook how
this division of labor serves to minimize technical error.

A second factor is operative on surgical services which also serves
to suppress the absolute number of technical errors: namely,
all requests for help are viewed as legitimate. When instructions for tasks are given, they are invariably followed by the tag
line, "If you run into any problems, give me a call." This statement is more than conversational filler; it is a reminder to subordinates that their superordinates are legally responsible for their
actions and are available to help. Further, the statement passes

on to the subordinate the responsibility of seeking help in situations beyond his level of competence. An important part of the subordinate's training is learning to discriminate between situations which he can and cannot handle. A request for aid is always honored. Two superordinate responses are common: (1) either the next person in the hierarchy performs the task himself, or (2) verbal instructions or pointers are offered. The first option is exercised when either time demands quick performance of the task, or when the task itself is seen as more complex than previously imagined:

> A myleogram [a diagnostic procedure involving the removal of spinal fluid and the injection of dye in the spinal column] was ordered for Mr. Eckhardt. A senior student was to instruct a junior student in the procedure. They tried without any success to get the needle in the proper space. After some fumbling and a few sticks at Eckhardt the senior student instructed the junior student to "get Paul." Paul came in and surveyed the situation. After examining Eckhardt's back he told the students, who were profusely apologizing for their failure, not to worry; that the problem was in Mr. Eckhardt's anatomy and not in their skills. He then proceeded with some difficulty to complete the procedure, instructing the students all the while (Able Service).

The skill of housestaff with such procedures helps establish their authority to students. The ease with which they place intravenous needles in the veins of the most troublesome patients is a very common way to impress students; it serves especially to humble senior students who are planning surgical careers and who are often competitive with first-year housestaff. The second option, verbal instructions and pointers, is exercised when, in the judgment of the superordinate, the task is not beyond the skill of the subordinate but rather the individual's lack of confidence in his own abilities is preventing task performance. Here, the subordinate is made to see that he can accomplish the task and at the same time he is offered support. Surgical housestaff learn to operate in much the same way that small children learn to ride bicycles. An unseen hand supports their efforts. The hand is withdrawn by stages and the novice finds himself operating on his own:

> Carl, the intern, was closing an incision while Mark, the chief resident, was assisting. Carl was ill at ease. He turned to Mark and said, "I can't do it." Mark said, "What do you mean, you can't? Don't ever say you can't. Of course you can." "No, I just can't seem to get it right." Carl had been forced to put in and remove stitches a number of times, unable to draw the skin closed with the proper tension. Mark replied, "Really, there's nothing to it"; and, taking Carl's hand in his own, he said, "The trick is to keep the needle at this angle and put the stitch through like this," all the while leading Carl through the task. "Now, go on." Mark then let Carl struggle through the rest of the closure on his own (Able Service).

Technical errors, then, are distributed throughout the surgical division of labor, but unevenly. More are made by beginners than the experienced. Technical errors do not damage an individual's claims to competence so long as he appears to learn from them and to make less of them over time. Supervision and the division of labor are arranged to keep such errors at a minimum.

Judgmental Errors

A judgmental error occurs when an incorrect strategy of treatment is chosen. These errors are also unevenly distributed through the division of labor. Subordinates who have only little discretionary power make few and relatively minor judgmental errors. Attending surgeons in charge of devising treatment plans make the most and the most serious judgmental errors. In these cases judgment is not always incorrect in any absolute sense; the surgeon, given the clinical evidence available at the time, may have chosen an eminently reasonable course of action, but the result—a death or complication—forces the surgeon to consider whether some alternative might have been more profitably employed. Clinical results, not scientific reasoning, determine how correct judgment is. Surgeons have an aphorism that expresses this: "Excellent surgery makes dead patients." By this they state most flat-footedly their understanding that textbook principles of care have to be compromised to meet the immediate situation, that results and not the elegance of a clinical blueprint separate acceptable from unacceptable practice.

The two most common judgmental errors that attendings make are (1) overly heroic surgery, and (2) the failure to operate when the situation demands. Overly heroic surgery involves the decision to operate when the patient cannot tolerate the procedure. This decision to operate is a surgeon's commitment to his skills; it is also a moral-ethical decision about what "tolerable" risk is and a decision about what the proper role of the physician is—whether he is charged with merely sustaining life or whether he may subject his patients to great risk in order to upgrade the quality of life. Needless to say, these are not easy or pleasant decisions. Consider the following:

> Mrs. Hardy is an old patient of Dr. Peters who has metastatic cancer. She has at most a few months to live. Recently her condition has worsened. Without an operation, she will probably literally vomit to death within a month. She has poor pulmonary and cardiac function; it is not clear whether she could tolerate an operation. If one is successfully performed, her life expectancy would be between three and six months— a month and a half of which would be postoperative convalescence (Able Service).

In this case can the surgeon justify putting a patient through the risk and trauma of surgery for such dubious rewards? But in good conscience can he stand idly by and sentence her to such an unpleasant death? An attending makes these decisions for himself. He may ask his subordinates what they would do if the decision were theirs. A favorite way of phrasing this question is, "What would you do if the patient were your mother?" After listening to his subordinates, the attending announces his decision. He need not justify this choice to other attendings. He need not explain the basis of his decision to his subordinates, although the didactic situation of surgical training encourages such explanations. To mobilize the resources necessary for action, the attending need only make up his mind. In this sense, his patients are his to do with as he wishes.

If subordinates disagree with an attending, there is very little they can do. A common tactic is to anticipate complications from a procedure and ask the attending how he intends to manage them:

> Mrs. Pratt is an obese woman with metastatic cancer on whom Dr. White has decided to perform an adrenalectomy and an oophorectomy [surgical removal of adrenal glands and the ovaries; an attempt to achieve a remission from cancer]. Mrs. Pratt's obesity and very poor pulmonary function make her a very poor operative risk. Both Mark and Paul seemed uneasy with White's decision. Mark told White that Mrs. Pratt would be like "a beached whale" following surgery and then he asked White a series of questions about the possibilities of embolism and the prophylactic measures White had in mind and about the difficulties of managing her pulmonary status following surgery. Paul then asked about gallstones and the possibilities of cholecystitis [inflammation of gallbladder]. After answering these objections, White left. Paul and Mark confided to each other that they felt uneasy about the surgery. Neither was certain that they would recommend it for their mother. Later, when I told Paul he seemed uncomfortable about the decision to operate, he replied: "Well, there is a great risk involved and it's not clear to me that the benefits are greater than chemotherapy, although White is right—the results of surgery can be absolutely dramatic, if you are lucky. Look—it's one thing for a patient to die from disease; you don't like it, but there's nothing you can do about it; you accept it. But for a patient to die because of something you did to him, because you gave him pulmonary edema [filling of lungs with fluid], or from a leaking anastomosis [seams that join resected body parts], that's a whole different thing. It makes you feel real bad when something you did kills somebody. It gives you pause for thought. Doctors aren't supposed to do that" (Able Service).

However, no matter how much they disagree with an attending's decision, no matter how much they grumble among themselves, subordinates defer to decisions with no more than polite questioning. The decision to operate is an apparently unchallengeable element in an attending's professional autonomy:

> I just make it a point not to disagree with attendings for two reasons. First, I'm not as smart as they are. And, second, the ultimate responsibility is theirs; and if they think that something should be done, I'll do it (Intern).

A second common judgmental error of attendings is the failure to establish a clear-cut plan of action for chronic problems. For most of these patients, secondary problems make operating impossible. These patients tend to linger in the hospital. They are not discharged nor are they aggressively treated. Often diagnostic tests reveal conditions in addition to the original problem requiring hospitalization. Each test in turn requires a further one. Intensive diagnostic studies are done on the patient even though he will not be extensively treated:

> Surgeons in general don't like theoretical or psychological problems. Things are either black or white. If they don't understand something, they try to put it out of their minds. For example, there are two patients on our service now whom we can't do anything with, and they really need something done. I think they will die without operations. But they are too sick to be operated on. The surgeon in this case gets frustrated and less aggressive. One of the worst things that can happen to a patient is to spend a long time on a surgical service. Surgeons lose interest in chronic problems. When the surgeon begins to lose interest, he starts asking for consultations, hoping that someone will take responsibility for the patient. Unfortunately some patients, not a lot, die because the surgeon loses interest (Chief Resident).

The error in judgment here need not express itself in a death or complication; surgical patients can spend considerable periods of time in the hospital, have little done for them, and be discharged without incident. Nevertheless, precious healing resources have been misallocated—a bed is taken up, time and effort are expended, and what the surgeon hoped to accomplish for the patient is never made certain. Moreover, such mistakes are more likely to be overlooked than others because they are not marked by an objective event such as death.

Though judgmental errors are most commonly made by attendings, some are also made by housestaff who have to make immediate decisions about patient management:

> Sam Jerome had his appendix removed on Baker Service. His postoperative recovery was anything but smooth. He was reoperated on for what was diagnosed as an obstruction but turned out to be an ileus [a condition where bowel has no peristaltic action]. Following the second operation, he developed a wound infection. Two days after the second operation, Brian, an intern, was sitting in the Baker conference room. I asked him how it was going and he replied, "Not so good. This responsibility can be devastating. It's just awesome. Take Jerome—I couldn't help thinking that the phenobarbital I ordered for him postop may have given him the ileus that caused us to think he was obstructed. That made us reoperate, and then he gets this wound infection" (Baker Service).

Housestaff routinely make such self-criticisms of their behavior, especially after deaths and complications. They review their entire course of action to see where they might have acted differently. Attendings encourage this reexamination of action and see it as symbolic of a subordinate's determination to learn:

> Until he is confident and secure, any good surgeon dreams about his operations. He reoperates, taking stitches in and out, revising his approach. He does this, too, for clinical situations. He rethinks how each patient was managed. This happens until he's secure. I did it. I expect my housestaff to do it. You need this kind of attention to detail, absolute dedication, and personal honesty to be a good surgeon (Attending).

Despite their claims of making serious and consequential judgmental errors, housestaff are not sanctioned for them for a number of reasons. First, they do not have the responsibility to make serious judgmental decisions; and, as Stelling and Bucher (1972) have shown for psychiatric and medical wards, one cannot be

accountable for an event unless one is also responsible for it.
Second, like technical errors, when quickly reported and infre-
quently committed, judgmental errors are seen as an inevitable
cost of training. They do not indicate that an individual is incompetent but rather they serve as evidence that he needs further
teaching. Judgmental errors, then, also reinforce a "training"
definition of the situation. Furthermore, as we shall see in chapter
4, there are structural limits placed on the housestaff's ability to
indulge in self-criticism. While social control of action rests on
self-criticism, the process of self-criticism itself is subject to social
controls.

Attendings are also somewhat insulated from the negative implications of their judgmental errors. First, their professional
accomplishments protect them from the imputation of defective
judgment: any individual failure must be weighed against many
successes, research publications, and the like. Second, operating
on difficult cases that others would not handle is a pride of place.
The attendings at Pacific pride themselves on their ability to treat
such cases. Death from judgmental error in such trying situations
is an uncomfortable fact of life:

> It would look suspicious if you are doing major surgery and,
> week after week, you have no deaths and complications.
> You're going to have these, especially deaths, if you do major
> surgery. You can lead a long and happy life without deaths
> and complications, but you have to give up major surgery
> (Attending).

There are times then when the surgical expectation of success is
waived. The reputation of the individual attendings of the surgery
department at Pacific and the reputation of the department itself
encourages heroic surgery in risky situations. In these cases, some
judgmental error is expected. These are not severely judged. Such
cases are seen not so much as mistakes but as a privilege and as a
burden of rank. Judgmental error in heroic situations—or operating too often in heroic situations—may earn an attending a
reputation among his colleagues and subordinates as a "matador," a "gunslinger," or "someone who sees a patient as just so

much meat on a table." Yet while such terms are indicative that the attending is not held in high esteem by his colleagues, being so labeled seems to have no noticeable effect on day-to-day behavior. It should also be noted that as a term of opprobrium there is a certain ambivalence involved in calling someone a "gunslinger" or a "matador." After all, in their respective cultures, such figures symbolize the heroic ideal. I suspect that most surgeons would rather be compared to Wild Bill Hickcock or Billy the Kid than to Caspar Milquetoast or Walter Mitty.

Normative Errors

A normative error occurs when a surgeon has, in the eyes of others, failed to discharge his role obligations conscientiously. Technical and judgmental errors are errors in a role; normative errors signal error in assuming a role. These errors are not distributed throughout the division of labor but are almost exclusively subordinate errors. Normative error occurs when, in the attending's judgment, a houseofficer's conduct violates the working understandings on which action rests. When a normative error occurs, the mistake renders it impossible to consider the person making it—in legal terms—a just and reasonably prudent individual. Viewed sociologically, normative errors challenge tacit background assumptions about how reality in a scene is constructed.

When spelled out, the background assumptions that govern clinical action are few, and they are drilled into the subordinate from his first clinical rotation as a medical student. The covering law for all behavior is, simply stated, "No surprises." Superordinates expect their subordinates to inform them of all changes, however small, in the service's status:

During the orientation meeting for the Able Service, Mark, the chief resident, explained what he expected during the next rotation: "If anything comes up, I want to know about it. I don't care what time it is; I want you to call. If there is a problem at four in the morning call at four in the morning.

Most likely, I'll listen to what you tell me and fall right back
to sleep. I may even forget that you called. But call. I don't
like to walk in here in the morning and find myself surprised
by what's going on in my service. I'm ultimately responsible
for what goes on here, so call me." He repeated this message
a number of times in a number of ways (Able Service).

The no-surprises rule is shared by all attendings. When interviewed, they all stated that the first expectation for housestaff
performance is compliance with the rule of no surprises. Interpreting the no-surprises edict is in actual practice a complex
decision for housestaff. Attendings dogmatically state the rule to
impress housestaff with its importance and to rescue everyone
from the technical and judgmental errors that are part of being
inexpert. Nevertheless, whether or not in any particular instance
to invoke the rule and call is a recurrent problem for subordinates. On the one hand, the housestaff member does not want to
look foolish, as if he cannot handle the simplest situations; and
on the other, he does not want to risk the attending's anger or the
patient's life should his assessment of the situation be incorrect.
Perhaps it needs to be pointed out that when a subordinate
chooses not to invoke the rule and does not call, he still risks the
attending's wrath even if he acts in a technically correct fashion.
At no time did I observe superordinates reacting negatively to
subordinates who called them for what later became unnecessary
reasons; and often what appears at the time as an unnecessary
reason appears retrospectively as very consequential:

Don, the senior student, at the end of a long and an eventful
day—there had been one unexpected death and one kidney
transplant—was talking with Greg, a junior student. "I called
Mark last night about Thelma Halsted [the unexpected
death]. It was four in the morning and he wasn't too pleased.
He told me to do what I would have done anyway. But the way
things worked out today, I'm really glad I called"
(Able Service).

Idealists may be dismayed that Don's reaction to an unexpected death is relief that he cannot be blamed. The more hard-

boiled and pragmatic will be grateful that from a personal tragedy, a moral lesson was salvaged and reinforced: when in doubt,
call, lest a death be your undoing. For the subordinate, calling is
always a safe strategy. Interpreting the no-surprises rule in the
framework of a zero-sum two-person game, a subordinate always
makes a game-correct decision to call. Yet subordinates feel that
there are costs attached to calling and may be under great pressure not to call because more than a correct response in an
interaction game is involved. In addition to the fear of looking
foolish, there is the desire to participate early in the intrinsic
gratifications of surgery, the belief that one learns from managing
new clinical situations, and a sense of dedication to the heroic
ideal that one is made or unmade by the quality of one's tests:

> The way you learn as an intern is by being put on the spot and
> coming through it. You develop a self-awareness that you can
> handle a lot of situations. The problem is learning what situa-
> tions you can't handle. There's a lot of pressure not to ask,
> a lot of fear of appearing foolish (Intern).

Despite these tensions and the resulting temptation for the subordinate to go it on his own, the no-surprises rule is the overarching
principle by which normative errors are defined.

We may ask, What is a surprise? The most correct answer is
anything that an attending chooses; and even though housestaff
occasionally feel that attendings apply no principles of selection,
attending behavior is more predictable than that. First, a surprise
for an attending is any violation of the principle of full and honest
disclosure. A surprise for the attending carries with it the implication that a housestaff member was lazy, negligent, or dishonest.
In practical terms, an attending finds himself surprised when he
discovers for himself something about a patient that housestaff
knew and neglected to tell him, or when he discovers for himself
something his housestaff should have known:

> I walked into the intensive care unit with Carl, Able's
> resident. Dr. White was on the phone. "I see a glucose value
> of 540," he grunts, and screws his face in an expression of
> pain. "Well, we were planning to operate today, but obviously

we've changed our thinking." White hung up and asked,
"What's this I hear about Thelma Halsted?" "I'm just getting
the story myself, sir," Paul, a second-year resident, answered.
"She had to be rushed to the Cardiac Care Unit for a pace-
maker. She's doing terribly," Carl volunteered. "Carl, why
wasn't I told?" Carl: "You were operating on the transplant,
sir." White: "That's no excuse. If you couldn't get away, you
could have called up to the OR and they would have tacked a
note on the door that I would have gotten the minute I
finished the case. That way, after surgery, I wouldn't stop
for coffee. I wouldn't stop and talk to people. Listen—when
one of my patients is dying, I don't like to be told by some
damn medical intern. I want to know what's going on with my
patients." White then wadded a piece of paper and threw it
across the nurses' station (Able Service).

Dr. Arthur was concerned that a complication from the
operation on Mrs. Prewitt might be a peroneal nerve palsy
[temporary paralysis of the foot from operative damage to the
peroneal nerve]. In clinic when he asked Ernest, the chief
resident, and Josh, the second-year resident, about it, they
both assured him that on morning rounds she was quite all
right. However, her examination on afternoon rounds revealed
a peroneal nerve palsy. Dr. Arthur's anger was apparent as we
left the room. We walked about sixty feet down the corridor
before he stopped to speak: "Goddammit! I will not have this
on my service. Do you understand? I ask if the patient has a
peroneal nerve palsy and am assured by my housestaff that
she doesn't and she damn well does. Now, this is not caused
by your not being smart enough to recognize the problem. It's
not your skill that is wanting here. This is a case pure and
simple of your being too lazy to get off your asses and look at
the patients. I will not tolerate this. Did you see this patient
this morning, Ernest?" "I did—yes, I did, sir." Arthur: "And
you didn't notice that she had no dorsal flexion [movement of
the foot at the ankle]?" Ernest: "No, sir." "Well, what the
hell were you looking at? What am I going to have to do to
get this service running right? If I can't count on my housestaff to provide decent preoperative and postoperative care
for my patients, then Grant and I will cancel our operations

until the patients we have are under control and until we are sure that we have housestaff who can do the job. Do I make myself clear?" (Baker Service).

Normative breaches are breaches of the etiquette governing the role relations between attending surgeons and housestaff. A normative error in turn carries with it the implication that a fundamental breach of etiquette governing the role relation between doctor and patient has occurred. When making decisions, the surgeon—any physician, in fact—is expected to bracket all systems of relevance to him as an actor in his other social roles and even bracket all systems of relevance to him in his other capacities as a surgeon. He is expected to treat conditions as they arise or to make certain that they will be treated before he moves on to other tasks. Fatigue, pressing family problems, a long queue of patients waiting to be seen, a touch of the flu—all the excuses that individuals routinely use in everyday life, are inadmissible on a surgery service. An attending who is surprised assumes that his housestaff have not been dispensing proper clinical care. Had they been, housestaff would have informed him of changes in clinical status.

Attendings are most frequently surprised by housestaff not keeping them abreast of unfolding events, but there are two other types of surprises that are treated as normative errors. A housestaff member's inability to get along with nurses is a failure that attendings treat as normative. It violates the tacit assumption that one will not let personality intrude on clinical care:

> After rounds, Arthur turned to Sharon, the head nurse of Baker Service, and asked: "Are there any nursing problems?" "Plenty!" Sharon replied. At Arthur's suggestion, we all went into the conference room to discuss it. Sharon explained that Dr. Carter and the nurses "didn't seem to get along this weekend." Arthur turned to Carter: "All right, Carter— what's the problem?" Carter explained: "Well, we had some problems getting a urinalysis done on Mrs. Yardley. The urine was collected but no one took it to the General Services Lab until I did at midnight. That's just one thing, but, really, the nurses on this floor are incredible. All the housestaff have

complained about it. The other night I was called every fifteen minutes. Once I was called because Crane's IV wasn't running. When I came down, I saw he had rolled over and kinked it. It was obvious that the night staff hadn't even looked at it." Arthur answered: "None of that bothers me. If you have to get up every fifteen minutes because nurses are too tired, lazy, or stupid, that's too bad for you, but it's what you're paid to do. You may even lose a pound or two. [Carter is overweight.] What bothers me is your fighting with staff. That accomplished nothing. In fact, it makes things worse. Look—you're a professional, you are better educated, better trained, and supposedly more mature than the staff. If you can't get along with them, we'll find someone who can. Do I make myself clear?" (Baker Service).

Housestaff failure to maintain good working relations on the ward is a serious mistake; it indicates that a subordinate lacks the skills necessary to run a surgical team. A housestaff member who quarrels with support staff is blamed—whatever the legitimacy of his complaint—for placing his own needs above those of patient care. There are ways of dealing with improper nursing; public quarreling is not among them. Further, as far as an attending is concerned, the problem with a subordinate who quarrels with nurses because they call too often for unnecessary reasons is that when he becomes a chief resident he may complain about his interns and that when he becomes an attending he may complain about his chief residents. This complaining may communicate that he is unavailable to help. In this case the whole set of controls built into task performance by the division of labor and norms of clinical care breaks down. Complaints about unnecessary work indicate to superordinates that a subordinate lacks the proper commitment.

A second serious error is similar to inability to work agreeably with nurses, that is, the inability to secure the cooperation of patients and their families. To housestaff fall the problems of obtaining informed consent, of gaining the patient's cooperation for preoperative and postoperative care—this is especially important because the involved patient can do much to prevent some postoperative complications, and of managing the anxieties of the patient and his family. A failure at any of these tasks is an indication that a subordinate cannot control the normal troubles of his environment. In addition, failure at any of these tasks creates extra work for attendings—these are unpleasant surprises—and all of this work is considered avoidable. It all stems from a subordinate not conscientiously filling his role. Technical and judgmental errors also create extra work, but such work is seen as an inevitable part of surgery. However, the extra work of normative errors is unnecessary. It is not viewed as an inevitable part of major surgery but as an inevitable consequence of minor surgeons.

Although normative errors are committed by both subordinates and superordinates, only those of housestaff are criticized and punished. Housestaff make normative errors because they are subject to so many cross-cutting systems of relevance that it is often impossible for them to bracket all systems of relevance, keep unfolding action under control, and avoid unnecessary problems for attendings. An intern or second-year resident's schedule is a grueling one: he works six and a half days, fifty weeks a year; a light working day is twelve hours; and at least two nights a week he stays in the hospital on call for emergencies. Given such working conditions, many other systems of relevance impose on the clinical one. There is the physiological one: housestaff need to eat and sleep. There is the social one: housestaff need time-out periods (this is an especially acute problem for married housestaff). There is the student one: housestaff need to study the problems they are treating. All of these are in addition to the multiple systems of the clinical role itself, which requires housestaff to coordinate treatment for as many as thirty-five patients, to provide a full complement of ancillary services, and to keep the ward running smoothly. Undoubtedly, trying to meet such multifocal demands explains to some degree why normative error occurs. Attendings, however, never allow such factors to excuse normative error. For them, there is no "good" excuse for a normative error because no other system of relevance is ever allowed ascendancy over the basic doctor-patient dyad and because normative errors are always interpreted as evidence that the houseofficer placed some other concern above patient care.

This is so despite the fact that normative errors such as quarrels with nurses or the failure to keep attendings fully informed need not result in outcomes that directly harm the patient. On the other hand, technical and judgmental errors always involve some discomfort to the patient yet are often interpreted as evidence of the individual houseofficer's commitment to clinical care.

Attendings escape blame for their normative errors for three reasons. First, the privileges of rank insulate them from many of the housestaff's cross-pressures. Because of their rank they are directly accountable to no one on a day-to-day basis. Second, membership in the American College of Surgeons, appointment to the Pacific faculty, and other credentials such as research publications and professional awards are a presumptive moral licensing. To be an attending at Pacific is to stand at the symbolic center of the value system of American medicine.[5] Basically, an attending is not publicly blamed for normative errors because there is no one to accuse him of such moral lapses. No one stands above him in the hierarchy and enforces the rule of "no surprises." The attending's position contrasts sharply with that of the houseofficer who has not yet been certified as morally fit to be a surgeon, whose commitments are now being tested. Third, although the attending is the legally responsible agent for patient care, the division of labor does not always reflect this. Generally attendings spend the greater portion of their time teaching or doing research rather than providing direct clinical care. Housestaff spend virtually all of their time providing direct care. Thus, division of labor itself frees the attending from the more prosaic responsibilities and pressures of patient care. All of these fall to housestaff, a fact which exposes them to concrete charges of normative failure. Rank, moral authority, and everyday task-structure insulate the attending and expose the housestaff to the danger of normative error.

Normative errors are taken seriously by housestaff and attendings. Housestaff fear normative error much more than they do technical and judgmental errors. They fear that normative errors destroy their credibility as responsible workers; they fear bad recommendations and other negative sanctions:

After he failed to inform Dr. White of Thelma Halsted's deteriorating condition and after White had reprimanded him, Carl left the room and sat dejected on a bench. He said: "That's it. I just blew two months' hard work in two minutes. It doesn't matter now what my work on the service was like. This is all he'll remember. It was a really dumb thing to do, a serious faux pas. I don't think she would have had any different care, really there was nothing White could have done about it. I guess it's just embarrassing for him to have a resident from another service tell him about his patients" (Able Service).

This fear of normative error on the part of housestaff runs deep and is shared by medical students. Among the students, we can see more clearly the logic-in-use that develops around performance and failure. Junior and senior medical students often state that the tasks they are assigned are so minor as to be worthless in evaluating their clinical skills. As a result, they think evaluations are based on their ability to be team members. Like housestaff, they are frightened of receiving recommendations that brand them as individuals who have difficulty respecting proper lines of authority. Interns and students both suffer the less rewarding aspects of their position in silence for fear of the repercussions of an overly noisy complaint:

Irv and Larry, the two students on Baker, have been dissatisfied with their stay on the service and were vigorously complaining to Christian, the intern, about it. Irv said: "It's not the amount of work, Chris—it's what we learn from it. We are not learning the principles of surgery and that's why we are here. What are we going to learn from anyway: doing the scut work or working-up a few patients and following through on them and reading about their problems?" Larry added: "Yeah, I don't mind being on call with the service because then you learn something. You work-up patients and see things. But to stay at the hospital just to change IV's—that doesn't make any sense." Chris answered: "Look—I didn't arrange the way that the service runs. If you have such complaints, if you feel this way, you should talk to Dr. Grant or Dr. Arthur." Irv replied: "C'mon, Chris. You know that we can't do that. We don't want a recommendation that says the student is unmotivated, uninterested in patients, and hard to work with. We want to work with patients, but we want to learn something, too" (Baker Service).

Attending reaction to normative error justifies housestaff's fear of these breaches. Attendings react strongly to normative error for a number of reasons. First, in the early stages of training, there are only minor variations in skill among subordinates. Normative performance is seen as an indicator of honesty and responsibility, two qualities that attendings feel subordinates must possess if they are to be capable colleagues:

> The most important thing is complete intellectual honesty, a willingness to admit problems and personal deficiencies. Someone who recognizes his errors and 'fesses up.' Look, I could teach a gorilla to operate in six months, but I can't teach honesty and responsibility. It's the people who have these qualities who make outstanding surgeons (Attending).

A technical or judgmental error then says something to an attending about a recruit's level of training; a normative error says something about the recruit himself. A second reason that normative breaches are so serious is that patients for whom attendings are legally responsible can be lost, without the attending's best effort being made on their behalf. A normative error then compounds the normal troubles of a surgeon's life. In addition to the inevitable deaths and complications, he must worry with those caused by personal as opposed to professional shortcomings; he is dealing with reducible error:

> Covering up is never really excusable. You have to remember that each time a resident hides information, he is affecting someone's life. Now in this business it takes a lot of self-confidence, a lot of maturity, to admit errors. But that's not the issue. No mistakes are minor. All have a mortality and a morbidity. Say I have a patient who comes back from the operating room and he doesn't urinate. And say my intern doesn't notice or he decides it's nothing serious and he doesn't catheterize the guy and he doesn't tell me. Well, this guy's bladder

fills up. There's a foreign body and foreign bodies can cause infections; infection can become sepsis; sepsis can cause death. So the intern's mistake here can cause this guy hundreds of dollars in extra hospitalization and it could cost him his life. All mistakes have costs attached to them. Now a certain amount are inevitable. But it is the obligation of everyone involved in patient care to minimize mistakes. The way to do that is by full and total disclosure (Attending).

A normative error breaches this system of full and open disclosure: this system protects attendings at the same time that it frees them for other activities. They need not be omnipresent if their housestaff keep them omniscient. The subordinate who fails here can expect severe punishments.[6] The rule of thumb attendings apply here is, even the most technically incompetent can be trained for something—he will rise or sink to his own level of proficiency. But the morally bankrupt represents a threat to the surgeons at Pacific and must be treated as a serious problem.

Quasi-normative Errors

Normative errors are breaches of standards of performance that all attendings share: quasi-normative errors are eccentric and attending-specific. Each attending has certain protocols that he and he alone follows. A subordinate who does not follow these rules mocks his superordinate's authority; his behavior is a claim that his judgment is as adequate as his superior's; and even though in no absolute sense can one claim that a mistake has been made, a subordinate who makes a quasi-normative error risks his reputation as a trustworthy recruit.

There are many decisions which surgeons are forced to make in the absence of scientifically established criteria. Great uncertainty surrounds much medical behavior.[7] From their own clinical experience and from medical journals, attendings marshal evidence to support one approach to a particular problem as opposed to another. However, the evidence is far from conclusive, debate continues, and a consensus fails to emerge. Some attendings approach a problem in one fashion with very good results;

others have equally good results with a competing approach. Despite the open-ended nature of the question "Which approach is better?", attendings in their everyday behavior can be quite dogmatic. Attendings believe that housestaff are on *their* services to learn *their* approach to the surgical management of disease. On other services, they can learn *other* approaches. Nevertheless, attendings are quite capable of making the theoretic distinction that separates quasi-normative from genuine error:

> First, you have to recognize that there are two different types of mistakes. There are genuine mistakes and there are mistakes of the "I don't do it this way; do it my way" variety. Those really aren't mistakes. At this hospital, for instance, take a patient with gastrointestinal bleeding. If he enters Dr. Arthur's service, Arthur wants to locate the source of bleeding. He performs an endoscopy [a procedure to view an internal organ; in this case the stomach is viewed through the mouth] on the patient, takes X rays, and maybe does an angiogram to locate the source of bleeding. Now, Dr. Henry doesn't think it's important to locate the source of bleeding. He places a nasogastric tube down the patient to suction any clots and get the stomach free of blood; he milks the stomach with an antacid bath; and if the bleeding stops, he doesn't care about the source. He figures if the bleeding doesn't stop, he still has time to do the tests to locate the source. One approaches the problem conservatively; the other, radically. Now these are both tremendously prominent men in the field. Who is to say that one way is right and the other is a mistake? (Attending).

In any actual case, the attending who is responsible for the patient's care is the one who says whether one approach is correct or not. The subordinate who favors and initiates another attending's approach over the one on whose service he is working opens himself up to severe criticism:

> On rounds, Dr. Arthur was examining the incision of Mrs. Anders, a young woman who had just received her second mastectomy. After reassuring her that everything was fine, everyone left her room. We walked a bit down the hall and Arthur exploded: "That wound looks like a walking piece of

dogshit. We don't close wounds with continuous suture on this service. We worked for hours giving this lady the best possible operation and then you screw it up on the closure. That's not how we close wounds on this service, understand? These are the fine points that separate good surgeons from butchers, and that's what you are here to learn. I never want to see another wound closed like that. Never!" Arthur then was silent, he walked a few feet, and then he began speaking again: "I don't give a shit how Dr. Henry does it on the Charlie Service or how Dr. Gray does it on Dogface; when you're on my service, you'll do it the way I want. There's no excuse for this, especially after I gave a little speech at Thursday's conference that I never use continuous sutures. If you work for me, you do things my way. I don't want any work screwed up by incompetent closures. Do you understand?" (Baker Service).

For the attending, more than professional pride is involved in quasi-normative errors: housestaff using their own independent judgment appear insubordinate to him. Compliance with attending dictates, however open to debate they are, is an indicator that a subordinate is a responsible member of the team who can be trusted. Attendings feel that the subordinate who makes quasi-normative errors is also likely to make normative errors: his behavior does not inspire trust:

The thing that offends me the most is when I tell someone they made a mistake and I give him my list of reasons— because he's always entitled to know why he is wrong—and then he tells me that it was okay, and that he was entitled to make a mistake for his own experience. When people put their own experience above patient care, I find it intolerable. Just the other day, I had a fourth-year student pull a nasogastric tube on the second day postop of a patient of mine. I told him that this was not wise. The patient had no bowel sounds nor had he had a bowel movement, and I take both as indications that a nasogastric tube is ready to be pulled— however, in this guy's judgment what he did was okay. He ignored my reasons. In fact, this guy's goal was not to be responsible for patient care but to be independent of higher-ups. He told me what he did was important for his own clinical development. He didn't give a fig about patient care. And nothing—nothing—nixes my confidence quicker than that. It's a privilege to learn here and the student is obligated to have a respect for our methods. They have to respect that the responsibility for the patient is ours; it's not the resident's patient—it's ours (Attending).

When a normative breach is made, a double error is involved: standards of clinical care are breached and the etiquette governing role relations among attendings and housestaff is breached. For quasi-normative errors, clinical care may be correctly administered and the general etiquette of role relations may even be followed—the subordinate may have informed his superior of the problem and been told to take care of it in the "usual" way. When a quasi-normative error is made, the subordinate is wrong for all the right reasons: his fault is that of *hubris*: he tried to act like an attending. Quasi-normative errors are idiosyncratic; behavior that would be formally correct on one service is not so on another. This is the cutting edge that distinguishes normative from quasi-normative errors: what counts as a normative breach is fairly constant from service to service. Nevertheless, attendings recognize each other's right to organize and run their services as they see fit; they hold that it is the subordinate's responsibility to accommodate himself to this state of affairs; and they agree that quasi-normative errors indicate that something is seriously awry with a subordinate.

The organization of work on a service determines how much room a subordinate will have for independent judgment and consequently how likely it is that he will make quasi-normative errors. On the Able Service, where supervision is relatively loose, subordinates have a great deal of room to maneuver and quasi-normative errors are relatively rare occurrences. On the Baker Service, supervision is relatively tight, subordinates have little room, and quasi-normative errors are more common. Housestaff when on the Baker Service state that they have to be "company men." Dr. Arthur has numerous personal eccentricities which he expects housestaff to respect and learn from. These express themselves in various eponyms: there are Arthur variations of operative procedures; there is the Arthur fluid-management regimen for postop care; and there is the Arthur method for managing gastrointestinal bleeding. Given the autocratic nature of surgical authority, the strong personal preferences of superiors are translated into absolute rules of conduct for subordinates. In everyday life, we label those with this power prima donnas: their own likes and dislikes become the rules others follow.

For their part, housestaff are eager to avoid quasi-normative errors. They fear finding themselves on an attending's wrong side, a state of affairs which can have devastating effects given the amount of control that attendings have over their careers. Often, the steps subordinates take to avoid quasi-normative errors can be amusing to the observer and sufficiently detached participant:

> Mark, Baker's chief resident, and Stan, a third-year resident, walked into Mr. Johnson's room on morning rounds. "Oh, my God! What's this?" they said in unison. "That's the patient with gastrointestinal bleeding I called you about last night," said John, the intern. "But you're treating him with an antacid bath," Stan said. "Sure! Isn't that the usual treatment? It's the way Henry does it on Charlie," said John. "You never treat gastrointestinal bleeding that way on Arthur's service. He'll blow his top if he sees this. We better get this out of here quickly," said Stan, all the while removing the antacid bath. As we left the room, Mark turned to me and said that a lot of surgery was foolishness and a lot of what surgeons believed was magic. But you couldn't argue with results (Baker Service).

More commonly, housestaff are not good-natured about meeting what seem to them the mere whims of superordinates; quasi-normative errors are a source of tension among housestaff and attendings. Housestaff resent that their judgment is not trusted; they feel that they are not given tasks commensurate with their skills; and they feel exploited as a cheap source of labor. Especially vexing to housestaff is the lack of debate and questioning that precedes many decisions:

> I don't like it when orders are given down from above without reasoning. I do not like decisions when there is no discussion. I realize that questions are not always appropriate; but when they are and you can't ask them, that makes things unpleasant. You can always ask some attendings why they are doing something, but you have to read the mood of others. It's all a matter of participation. When you are taken as a colleague, it is very pleasant; but when you are there just to carry out orders and to do the work, then I don't like it (Intern).

Housestaff also feel defenseless against the whims of attendings. They know that there is nothing they can do in the face of an attending's anger. They know that there is nothing they can do when attendings make errors, save talk among themselves. This inequality is, in fact, in one way or another one of their favorite topics of talk. Interestingly enough, it is not the amount of room itself which determines housestaff resentment of attendings. Housestaff can accept very narrow limits if they respect an attending's judgment and skill and if they feel they are learning despite eccentricities that must be tolerated. They then speak of the attending's behavior giving the service "color." On the other hand, housestaff may find relatively more freedom chafing if they do not respect an attending's judgment and if they feel that they are not learning much from a service. This finding parallels Goss's (1961) that professional expertise determines how well or poorly advice is received. Competent professionals need not pull rank since they can persuade by reason.

> Now, when you're on Arthur's service, you don't mind too much the way decisions are made. You know Arthur is such a good clinician that even though he's dogmatic, you believe him because he's usually right and when you disagree, you're usually wrong. But with Steele, you argue more because his opinions are not always sound, he makes wrong judgments in the operating room, and his clinical judgment is often poor. Your argue more—it's easier to argue—but since he is less secure, you have less leeway. He's always confused; and when you disagree with him, you feel he is probably wrong (Chief Resident).

On Baker Service, we were having coffee after morning rounds. Josh was talking about working with different attendings: "It's really funny. When Arthur speaks, it's as if he has a pipeline from God himself—he's that sure that what he says is right and the only way to treat a patient; and you don't think to question him. Then, when you're on Charlie Service, Henry will tell you with equal conviction an exactly opposite way of doing things. And when he says it, you believe him" (Baker Service).

Quasi-normative errors are serious mistakes for subordinates to make; for them to damage a subordinate, however, he must make them on more than one service or he must make them blatantly (see chapter 5 for a fuller discussion). Housestaff are forgiven an error or two that may reflect a lack of familiarity with a service. In fact, strong reactions of attendings to these errors is a way they communicate to housestaff how seriously they take their personal rules. It is a way of showing what the proper alignment of roles is, of communicating to housestaff that they are in the hospital not so much to treat patients as to learn to treat them. Attendings acknowledge that the system is one in which it is difficult to be a subordinate:

Surgery is a funny business: You force strong-willed, aggressive, intelligent individuals to become peons. The goal is by having these individuals sublimate all their own independence, they will come out five years later as strong individuals with confidence in their own skills, judgment, and ability (Attending).

Exogenous Sources of Failure

Surgical intervention also fails for a number of reasons that do not implicate the competence of the surgeon in any direct way. The surgeon's strong sense of individual responsibility has him turn to these reasons only when the search procedure fails to reveal any physician error or when the reason is glaringly obvious. These labels for failure are then a residual category. They raise no questions of physician competence, deviance, and the social control of performance.

First, there is *failure from disease.* Sometimes the best efforts of surgeons cannot cure those in the more advanced stages of terminal illness. Operative complications always raise questions about the adequacy of surgery; but deaths, especially when separated from the operation by a respectable period of time, do not terribly threaten surgeons. These deaths indicate to surgeons what the limits of their skills are; and they are seen as inevitable. Much disease is irreversible. An interesting feature of the allocation of effort on a surgery ward is the division of patients into two classes: salvageable and nonsalvageable. Heroic care goes only to salvageable patients. The nonsalvageable do not receive emergency cardiac resuscitation or other aggressive life-prolonging measures. This is not to say that the surgeons at Pacific practice euthanasia; rather they limit their heroism. Nonsalvageable patients are allowed to die from their diseases and not saved to suffer from them. These patients are still treated—they are not ignored—but the surgeon does not play all his cards. Salvageable patients are candidates for heroic measures. These two classes of patients help determine the allocation of scarce healing resources.

Second, there is *patient procrastination* or *noncooperation.* Often surgical intervention fails because patients neglect to report symptoms until too late. This happens for a variety of reasons. They may read the symptom correctly and fear the cure —women with breast cancer, for example. They may have religious beliefs that inhibit medical intervention—Christian Scientists, for example. They may not have easy access to health care by virtue of being poor or uninsured. Surgeons view these patients with a mixture of incredulity, compassion, and disgust. Also, patients may report symptoms, consent to care, and then balk at proposed cures—patients facing amputations are an example. These patients refuse to consent to the more radical treatments offered them and agree only to procedures more limited than what the surgeon desires. Here, the surgery performed is a compromise between what the surgeon thinks he can get away with and what the patient will accept as necessary.

On Able Service, Mark and I had left the room of a patient
who had refused to consent to a procedure that White thought
best—a below-the-knee amputation and a dissection of the
lymph nodes in the groin. Despite Mark's best efforts—he
appealed to the patient's responsibility to his family, to his
youthful appearance, and the greater promise for a vigorous
life the more extensive procedure promised, and claimed that
the operation was not as bad as the patient feared—the
patient refused to hear any of it: "You can cut to here and
no further," he said, drawing an imaginary line across his
knee with his hand. When we left the room, I asked Mark if
such refusals were common. He answered: "It happens. It's
rare but it happens. When it happens, I try to explain to the
patient why we want to do the procedure we do. I mean, I
really try to explain so that he understands. I never try to
bullshit somebody into an operation. And then if he still
refuses, I try to work out some compromise that the patient
and I can live with. Now, take this guy: he might be right to
gamble. If I were in his place, I'd accept the knee amputation
and the groin dissection. But I can't say for sure that the
lymph nodes are the source of his problem so I can't in good
conscience play God and demand he have the fuller operation.
He may be right—who knows? As a surgeon, I can't put a gun
to his head and demand that he have what I think is the best
operation" (Able Service).

Here, the patient must share responsibility for the outcome with
the surgeon. The necessity for "informed consent" often com-
promises what the surgeon would like to do.

Third, there is *nursing and support staff error*. Often failure
can be traced to the mistakes of nurses and others involved in
direct patient care. Medication fails to get passed properly; intravenous solutions are not replaced on time, or they are run in too
fast or slow; tests are scheduled but fail to get carried out; blood
samples are contaminated; dressings are not changed promptly
and wounds are not kept clean enough—the list is endless. On the
one hand, subordinates are responsible for seeing that nurses are
mobilized and that work gets done properly; but, on the other
hand, housestaff cannot be responsible for everything everyone

does. So housestaff are held accountable for nursing error that emerges from creating tension with nurses, and they are held accountable for not properly dealing with nursing error. Normal nursing errors are treated by doctors as difficulties in a different chain of command. They are reported to the appropriate authority, and it is assumed that nurses will keep their own house in order.

Fourth, there is *machine malfunction.* Some failures occur because of breakdowns in the enormous technology that supports care in the modern hospital. Computers print out the wrong values for diagnostic tests; ventilators fail; pumps fail. Such things happen, and there is little the surgeon can do, save have the offending machinery replaced or repaired. Failure does not threaten the claim to competence. However, for novices the breakdown of machinery can pose a real threat to confidence. The inexperienced may connect the failure of the machine with a failure of their own skills since they do not have enough practice to form a sense of mastery at the task. The recruit may even feel that the machine is trying to tell him something.

three

Routine Surveillance as Social Control

The typology of error discussed in chapter 2 is an observer's scheme for categorizing how surgeons explain, control, and correct failure. The observer's typification is inadequate in two ways. On the one hand, the typification scheme of surgeons is more subtle. There are many specific varieties of the general type, technical and judgmental errors. There are preoperative, intraoperative, and postoperative techniques and judgments; and each of these is capable of further subdivision so that intraoperatively, for example, surgeons speak of intubating, preparing and draping, opening, clearing the field, making the correction, closing, and extubating as distinct stages of an operation—each with its own set of techniques and judgments and its own calculus of success and failure. On the other hand, the typification scheme of surgeons is more gross. There is only one critical distinction superordinates make in evaluating a failure: was the failure the result of someone doing what any reasonable person in the scene might have done, or was it the result of less than responsible behavior? Error is a dichotomous category. Now, to say that error is both a dichotomous category and a category capable of multiple subdivisions is to say that there is a qualitative difference among errors. Two categories, technical and judgmental, sustain a definition of the situation as normal. Given the necessity for actors to learn by doing, the "surgery is a body-contact sport" philosophy that attendings share with varying degrees of intensity, a mistake assigned to these categories is accepted as routine and inevitable and treated as an occasion for passing on the tricks of the trade. Two categories, normative and quasi-normative, suspend normal definitions of the situation. These are extraordinary errors that challenge the tacit assumptions that make social order possible. A mistake assigned to these categories is treated as a moral breach by a responsible agent and as an occasion for corrective remedies, the most immediately available being the "talking-to" (Freidson and Rhea 1972).

Chapter 2 provides several examples of talking-tos delivered at the time the infraction was discovered. This sanction is so immediately available because it requires an attending physician to mobilize nothing save his outrage. He need not win the approval of his colleagues nor satisfy the requirements of due process nor marshal any evidence beyond what the scene makes immediately available to sustain his claim.

Housestaff report that they find these public talking-tos humiliating; that they make them feel "really worthless"; and that the fear of being a victim motivates performance. At the same time this fear creates bitterness and resentment toward attendings. The mixture of awe and ill will directed at attendings emerges as a common theme in autobiographical accounts of medical training. Especially good examples are found in Cook (1972), Nolen (1970), Glaser (1973), Viscott (1974), and Dr. X (1965).

My cataloging of error in chapter 2 is too taxonomic to give an adequate understanding of the processes by which superiors assign mistakes to one category or another, typify subordinates as responsible or not, and regulate the quality of performance. A taxonomy of mistakes does not reveal the judgmental work done by actors in the scene to construct a reality. In this chapter I hope to remedy that defect. The routine surveillance of action during rounds is the major mode of everyday social control. Rounds are also the least public control as they involve only an attending and his subordinates. Mortality and Morbidity Conferences (see chapter 4) involve an assembly of attendings and subordinates. Promotion decisions (see chapter 5) involve the collegium of attendings. Since rounds serve as the major mode of everyday social controls, it is then that the judgmental work of actors is most apparent. For our purposes three recurring dimensions of rounds behavior are noteworthy: the tension between rule by clinical experience and rule by scientific knowledge; the questioning process; and the place of horror stories in the oral culture of medicine.

Rounds Behavior

There are three different types of rounds that surgeons employ to monitor their performance—work rounds, chart rounds, and attending rounds. Participants in the scene identify at least three other types of rounds. First, there are card rounds, a shortened form of chart rounds. These are a review of a patient's medication. They are often instigated by nurses when prescriptions become outdated and medications are not needed or cannot be dispensed by them legally. As such, card rounds are a nursing control on physician behavior. Second are "chief resident rounds." Alternative terms are used by others, but whatever the designation these are a quick run through the patients with one eye on the clock. Here quickness is the key. (The goal is to reach home before one's children are asleep.) Third are coffee or nutritional rounds. These are held in the cafeteria and usually focus on any and everything, save patients.

Work Rounds

Work rounds are a method for organizing work and allocating effort, as well as checking progress. As a rule, they occur twice daily: like opening and closing exercises in grade school, they are the first and last group projects of the day. On work rounds, subordinates alone participate. In the morning, they decide on what needs to be done that day and they divide the work among themselves. The patients on the service are divided between junior and senior medical students, with interns sharing the load in especially heavy periods. The students have responsibility for completing the most routine work on patients; they are expected to get to know their patients as well as possible in a biomedical sense, but they are also expected to know them well enough as social beings to spot any problems that will interfere with recovery. Medical students are often told by their teachers to get to know patients now because they will never again be in a position to spend so much time with them. To this students reply that it's a shame that the time in their career when they are around the most is the time when they can do the least. All of this routine work is called "scut." The acronym is ironically explained as "some clinically useful training." More complex tasks are reserved for housestaff. Even still, housestaff complain that an inordinate amount of their effort is wasted on tasks beneath their abilities. On afternoon rounds, subordinates regroup, evaluate the results of the day's tests, decide what work is necessary that evening, and reserve the tasks that can wait for the next morning. Also, on afternoon rounds, some extra care is usually made to answer patient questions. The press of a day's work prevents this on morning rounds, which the service rushes through in order to arrive on time at their first appointments.

During work rounds, subordinates are not critical of each other's performance. A joking reproach is the strongest rebuke I ever observed. Housestaff are concerned to make sure that all work is done, that any special requests of the attending have been carried out, and that no troubles have developed that they are unaware of. Improperly done work, missed assignments, and scheduling mix-ups are all seen as group problems. They are everyone's concern and no one's fault. Responsibility for the work of the service is corporate. Nevertheless, this corporate feeling is subject to great strain. There are several factors that predispose attendings to blame junior housestaff for problems. A student is seen as too inexperienced to have major responsibility. A chief resident is too experienced and trustworthy. In addition, attendings have invested five years in a chief resident's training and are committed to believing in his excellence. This leaves interns and second-year residents in the most exposed position, most vulnerable in bad times. In addition, despite the ideal of corporate responsibility, housestaff fear that their colleagues, when confronted by attendings for questionable behavior, will try to shift the blame. They fear being made scapegoats for tasks that fall outside their responsibility:

> There are two ways people make it in academic medicine.
> You can do it on your own ability or by negating the ability of
> others. Too many guys are obsessed with finding a way out.
> You know, saying it's not really my patient or I wasn't on

call last night or something like that. Or they'll go back and find an abnormal lab value in some old test and then argue that it [the death or complication] was happening all along and their decisions were not what did it (Intern).

Josh and the rest of the Baker Service gathered in the conference room after being dressed down by Arthur for shoddy performance. Arthur claimed that the kindest thing that could be said about their work was that it was "disinterested" and the strongest that it "borders on criminal malpractice." All of the service felt that nothing they had done justified such an outburst. They all commented on this. One of the junior students regretted that Ernest, the chief resident, had missed rounds because he would have known how to handle Arthur; the student expressed the hope that when Arthur spoke with Ernest, the chief resident would be able to explain things and straighten things out. Josh Carter, the resident second-in-command, answered, "Fat chance! Don't bet on it. No, Ernest will tell Arthur that he's been letting me run the service. Yeah, I bet that's what he tells him. You'll see, I'm the one who's going to wind up getting screwed" (Baker Service).

Despite this fear of being made a scapegoat, it is rare in actual practice. In fact, as the text below makes clear, a very real opposite danger exists that problems cannot be shifted to those to whom they rightfully belong. One reason is that attendings do not accept such accounts as legitimate:

Forget the resident who says, "I don't know what happened—it was my night off." He'll never make it. I say that in the army there were only three answers you could give: "Yes, sir"; "No, sir"; and "No excuse, sir." That's true for surgery, too (Attending).

For attendings, the way that subordinates divide work is immaterial; quality performance is demanded; and lapses are everyone's responsibility. Because of this, attendings do not believe that housestaff can be asked unfair questions about actions taken on the service. A response that denies responsibility or knowledge is unacceptable for it communicates to attendings a disinterest in clinical care.

Work rounds are then a method that subordinates employ to protect themselves as a corporate group. This activity guarantees that each member of the service will see each patient daily, regardless of his individual responsibility for the patient.

The information exchanged during rounds is a capsule summary of the salient facts of a patient's clinical history. The informal division of labor has members of the service take turns assuming primary responsibility for patients admitted to the service. This random method of matching patient and subordinate is seen as the most equitable way of distributing both "scut work" and interesting cases. The rule of assignment, "Your turn—your patient," is interpreted in much the same way as the rule of assignment in a welfare office that Zimmerman (1970) discusses, both in its application and in its breach. If a service member feels he has an oversupply of cases that are purely scut, he may request a patient whom he feels is interesting; or if a service member feels an embarrassment of riches with regard to interesting cases, he may volunteer for a patient ill with an uninteresting disease. The member of the service with responsibility for the patient according to the informal division of labor among subordinates recites the following: when the patient is new and has not yet been introduced to the service, the patient's initial complaint and proposed plan of treatment; and, once the service knows a patient, his medications and their indications; the latest lab reports, with a special emphasis on important or abnormal lab values, the plan and schedule of treatment for the patient, and any other relevant and unusual information about the patient, such as dietary restrictions or secondary problems.

Basically, work rounds circulate the information that everyone who treats the patient should know to the entire group of subordinates. Work rounds provide a patient with ongoing treatment and they allow housestaff to be in command of the situation. They rehearse leadership and decision making. They also rehearse attending rounds which are, as we shall see, a competence test. In surgical training, in all clinical education, the patient is the subject matter which must be mastered. Work rounds are a group review session. Medical education is in some sense a paradigm of an open classroom, at least in its clinical aspects. On the service first- through seventh-year students are working at tasks, mastering them, and then moving on to tasks of greater complexity. Further, it is often the individual who has recently learned who passes on his newfound knowledge. This idyll of self-learning suffers some tensions. Some individuals feel they progress too slowly. Sometimes discussion passes over the heads of the least experienced; other times it cannot sustain the interest of the most experienced. Always, there is the problem of overload. The peer network that evolves is not unlike the one that Bossert (1975) describes for third- and fourth-graders in open classrooms.

Chart Rounds

In addition to work rounds, housestaff prepare themselves for attending rounds and monitor their own work by chart rounds. Here, housestaff review a patient's medical records. Chart rounds serve a number of purposes. First, they allow housestaff to trace the natural history of disease processes. Second, they provide a quick and efficient way of keeping up to date on a patient's condition without ever seeing the patient. From the chart, the housestaff member can often glean all the information about patients necessary for his purposes at hand. In fact, housestaff comment that really good charting and nursing makes their actually seeing patients unnecessary.

> Ernest and I were heading for the Intensive Care Unit to see Mr. Grotesk, a patient who had had a cardiac arrest the night before. As we were talking down the corridor Ernest said to me: "The thing about the ICU is that when you get a really good nurse, you never have to see the patient. You can ask a few questions about blood gases, vital signs, and urine output, read the chart, and look at a few numbers and you'll know everything you need to know" (Baker Service).

Third, in cases where little progress has been made, service members use chart rounds to search for new clues to an illness that they have not yet understood. Fourth, and most important, chart rounds are a way housestaff have of checking the thoroughness, skill, understanding, and reliability of the medical students

on the service. The major part of the student's responsibility
consists of charting the findings from the patient's physical
examination. The student's clinical impressions are written up
and added to the patient's record. For the student, this is practice
in diagnosis. The student's results are then checked by a member
of the housestaff, who repeats the examination of the patient for
himself. Housestaff use chart rounds to monitor the performance
of students. Part of the review is of the actual clinical findings
and part of it is of the art of chart writing. Since so much medical
communication is in this medium, the second part of this review
is not unimportant. Charts provide a running record of subordinate performance. However, we never observed attendings in-
dexing poor performance by a retrospective reading of charts.
Nevertheless, as Freidson and Rhea (1972) point out, the clinical
record is always latently supervisory.

Attending Rounds

Attending rounds occur at the pleasure of the attending: on the
Able Service, this was once a week; on the Baker Service, it was
three or five days a week. The attendings of the other two surgical
services made more rounds than the attendings of Able but less
than those of Baker. These rounds are the occasion when patients
are visited by attendings, when the lessons of clinical experience
are passed on, when a pretense of discussion before decision
making is provided, and when attendings match their own clinical impressions against those of their housestaff and, in cases of
discrepancy, seek accounts. Made to do different work for different people—they provide reassurance and comfort for patients, teaching for students, colleagueship for housestaff, and a
stage for attending performances—these rounds have a strong
social control component. Attending rounds are, if nothing else,
a poking around on the part of superordinates to make certain
that their houses are kept in order. When the service is running
smoothly, the teaching, collegial, and humane work of rounds
can be accomplished. That is to say, these tasks are attended to
only when social control is unnecessary or completed. The social

control component of rounds is usually routinely disposed of.
I did notice in those cases where this was not so that attendings
did not lessen patient contact; if anything, they expanded it. Perhaps they felt that if their housestaff were not doing things right,
then *they* would have to do everything. Because clinical dialogue
is so embedded in the environment, the testlike quality of rounds
is sometimes lost on participants. The way social control is built
into rounds allows for less threatening definitions of reality than
competence testing.

Attending rounds are governed by a formal etiquette that gives
their enactment a ceremonial flavor. First, the members of the
service file into the patient's room in order of rank: attendings
followed by housestaff in order of years of experience followed by
students. The exit pattern is the same. The only variation in this
ritualized coming and going is minor and is a function of the very
human problem of fitting so much human traffic through such a
narrow space as a doorway.[1] At any rate, this traffic pattern never
varies with regard to attendings. They are always the first in and
the first out. Next, if an attending has never met a patient before,
the houseofficer who is responsible for the patient introduces him
in a stylized fashion:

"Dr. X, meet Mr. Morris. Mr. Morris is a fifty-two-year-old
male who was admitted with a possible gastric ulcer. His vital
signs are good. His chemistries are not yet back from the
lab. We have scheduled a small bowel series for tomorrow
and a large bowel series the day after that."

The attending then shakes hands with the patient, asks him a few
questions, makes a quick physical exam, and assures the patient
he can help him. Attendings state that this laying on of hands is
as much for the patient's benefit—to satisfy his expectation of
what doctors do—as for anything the doctors hope to learn.
Moreover, cheerful assurance is only one of a number of possible
interaction styles. It is the one attendings of both the Able and
Baker Service preferred. An alternative style that has been discussed is "hanging crepe" (Siegler 1975). When an attending
hangs crepe, he paints a hopeless case and offers only mild hope

that he can salvage the situation. There is, I think, reason to believe that there is a positive bias in surgeons' interaction styles. Partly this is a denial of the possibility of failure. Partly this is a device to mobilize the patient's healing resources and cooperation. The surgeon who told his patient, "Good God, I don't think you're going to make it. I just hope you don't die on the table" would win neither friends nor awards for his bedside manner. The importance of individual action predisposes surgeons to aggressive confidence more than other physicians who are not so personally committed to their interventions and who are more tolerant of the natural course of disease. If an attending has met a patient, he asks him a few questions and then turns to his subordinates. He asks the group questions about patient care and about recent literature bearing on the patient's condition. The person who has responsibility for the patient is expected by the group to field these questions. Occasionally, attendings will direct questions to particular individuals, especially when their performance is suspect.

If all questions put to housestaff are answered satisfactorily and if things appear in order, then knowledge of good performance builds. Housestaff become trusted. In the future, more time on rounds is spent teaching and being collegial with subordinates. If things appear awry and housestaff cannot explain why, attendings spend greater time on the social control of performance. Housestaff are not trusted. The distrust of subordinates is a consequence of the way they acquit themselves on rounds:

> You look at the way patients are approached. You try to find out if your housestaff know what's going on. Say Mrs. X has been a patient for three days and you ask about Mrs. X's chest X ray and they haven't seen it. Then you feel that they don't know what's going on. Or say Mrs. X has been in a lot of pain and they don't know about it. You don't expect your young people to know all the answers to all the problems; but you expect them to know what the problems are. You expect them to know what is happening and why. When you find they don't, you begin to check things more closely. You look

at the dressings to see if they are bothering themselves with keeping them clean (Attending).

Stelling and Bucher (1972) have defined the zone of autonomy that surrounds subordinates as "elastic"; that is to say, monitoring and performance covary. Quite clearly, monitoring is related to the evaluation of performance; indeed, monitoring itself may be a deviance-amplifying mechanism (see Wender 1968). It is deviance-amplifying because when an attending feels the need to increase monitoring he is already convinced that something is wrong. What is wrong are the signs that housestaff are not getting the job done. Attendings notice, for example, that wounds are not dressed properly; that scheduling problems are developing and that tests are not being done; that lungs are not cleared vigorously enough following surgery; or that women are not made to exercise their arms following mastectomies. The attending then surveys patients more intensively and questions housestaff more closely and more often about the actual quantity of their effort as opposed to the theoretic quality of that effort. In such cases, the attending is more likely to find errors. Those that he finds he is more likely to brand as normative or quasi-normative. He finds them because he is looking for them and because he is sure they are there for the finding. On the other hand, when the attending feels that the service is in order, the questions he raises are limited and confined to the theoretic justification for action. In this case an attending finds technical and judgmental errors; he finds these because at least for the moment his housestaff are above suspicion of more serious breaches.

A consequence of this pattern of surveillance is that during periods of high monitoring, housestaff often feel that they are being unfairly treated by attendings. Their resentment of their subordinate and defenseless position grows, and they begin to form assessments of attendings as capricious, arbitrary individuals who are impossible to please or understand:

The members of the Baker Service were complaining about their most recent dressing-down by Dr. Arthur. Josh Carter was visibly upset; he sat apart from the group and chain-

smoked. Darwin, the senior student, offered him support:
"Look. You know with Arthur it takes only one thing to go
wrong for him to jump up and down all over you. And once he
finds something, he nit-picks until he finds a whole raft of
things. Maybe if Jerome's wound hadn't been shut and with
paper tape at that, then maybe we would have made it."
(Using paper tape on the Baker Service is a quasi-normative
error.) This prompted the junior student who had mistakenly
taped the wound shut to apologize to Carter. Carter replied,
"It's okay, really it is. If the wound hadn't been taped shut,
then he would have found something else. Really, it's not
your fault. If it hadn't been this, it would have been
something else. That son-of-a-bitch is just a malevolent bastard" (Baker Service).

The housestaff perception that the attending was just looking for
something to complain about is correct but it is also incomplete.
Housestaff neglect to explain why the attending would be motivated to look for something to begin with. For their part,
attendings look for problems because, following their rule of "forgive and remember," they discern a pattern in the work around
them and failures can no longer be considered random clinical
events. So the fact that without advance warning attendings step
up monitoring, become more dogmatic about the way they want
work done, and more critical of subordinates is not arbitrary. It
may appear so to the subordinate who is not aware that an
attending has changed his interpretation of a subordinate's performance from favorable to unfavorable and reread past events
in this light. The subordinate is after all doing what he has done
all along and this has always been acceptable in the past.

Moreover, there is a predictable temporal patterning to the
surveillance of performance on a rotation. At first, monitoring is
rather complete as the attending lays down the law in the beginning. He defines his expectations for subordinate performance.
Then, the attending withdraws somewhat. If things go well,
surveillance relaxes and at the end of a rotation, housestaff-
attending relations are relaxed and cordial. However, if things go
poorly, then the attending steps in again and provides tighter

control. In such cases at the end of a rotation, relations among housestaff and attendings are strained, highly formal, and very unequal:

> When you have problems with an attending, they will declare themselves at the end of a rotation and they are really a matter of no longer communicating with an attending. Of course, attendings bawl you out, humiliate you—that's part of training. Some, however, go beyond that. They order too many tests; they make too much work; they show poor judgment in the operating room. When that happens, it's best to stay away from them as much as possible (Chief Resident).

But it is precisely at this point that the attending is most difficult to avoid because this is when he is paying the most attention to work. He may not appear any more often—Dr. Peters never makes rounds more than once a week—however, the time spent is more intense; the attending spends more time asking questions about each patient and he spends more time getting clinical readings of his own. As a consequence, the attending has more direct orders to give. Furthermore, to the extent that the attending takes charge of a patient's care, a subordinate has his autonomy usurped.

Clinical Experience vs. Scientific Reasoning

It is through a system of such give-and-take that attendings evaluate housestaff, regulate performance, and identify deviant housestaff—those who cannot meet the demands of a surgical career. The power of the attending is most noteworthy. On the basis of his observations on rounds, however hastily they might be made, the superordinate encroaches on the autonomy of subordinates by countermanding orders and reproving behavior. In the process, careers are made and broken. This almost total control of action in the scene is a power and privilege of rank. As judgmental and quasi-normative errors indicate, the word of the attending is law. The attending may not always be right; but in cases where he finds himself disagreeing with his housestaff, he need not give good reasons for his preferences. To have them acted out, he need only announce them. On the other hand, the good reasons of a subordinate are in themselves never a sufficient cause for attendings to embark on a course of action. This is to say, that in disputes over what a clinical reality is, the attending has the last word. He has the right to construct reality as he sees fit. The subordinate is compelled for all practical purposes to accept this definition of reality, however much he may resent it, distrust it, or disagree with it. This power of the attending to construct the binding interpretation of reality has powerful control implications. It means that the attending whose professional behavior is improper is beyond the reach of any subordinate who notices it. Subordinates' notions of the justice of a system of professional control rests on the faith that such behavior cannot long remain secret and in time other attendings will know of and be forced to act on this guilty knowledge. At the same time, houseofficers themselves are defenseless against whatever charges an attending may level. The completion of their own training rests on the hope that attendings will be tolerant and forgiving of their errors. In this situation the power of an attending and its restraint are striking. In rounds behavior, we are able to see what beliefs legitimate this power, what beliefs restrain it, and what tensions underlie it. There are two competing systems of legitimation for medical authority: clinical expertise and scientific evidence.[2] These systems are not of equal importance: in the case of discrepant opinions, arguments based on clinical expertise override those based on scientific evidence.[3] Such a system of legitimation concentrates power in the person of the attending. On the one hand, he is the active creator of the most recent scientific evidence; in some specific cases the attending is literally the last word on a subject. On the other hand, by virtue of his clinical experience, he knows when scientific findings are not appropriate for charting a course of action. He knows the rules and their exceptions. The subordinate is learning the rules; he does not yet have enough experience to recognize the exceptions.

Rule by scientific evidence alone implies a more egalitarian and formally rational legitimation of authority; and as a consequence, a more formally rational task-structure. Ironically, this mode of legitimation alone is both less collegial and more egalitarian. In such a system, all arguments have equal weight; the authority of evidence and the authority of the person who presents it are independent. Subordinates who read widely are in a position to challenge an attending's authority and increase their own autonomy. Thus, those in the training situation would have more equal access to the source of legitimate authority. However, because of the greater importance of clinical expertise, superordinates are in a position to reject scientific evidence that they feel violates their own sense of what the situation requires:

> We were visiting Mr. Darnell, who had a proctocolectomy [removal of rectum and distal end of colon with externalization of proximal colon] the day before. As Arthur was surveying the wound, Ernest asked him about a new technique developed by Dr. Stanley and reported in a recent journal article. According to Ernest, Stanley reported that on a series of patients using this new technique, he had no instances of a particular complication. Arthur replied: "I've tried that technique and I've seen patients on whom it was used, and I'm convinced it's not a bit better." Ernest repeated: "But in a large series, there were no complications." Arthur answered: "Then Stanley has a poor memory, or he didn't include in his series at least six of his patients I treated for that complication." Ernest asked: "Doesn't that call for a letter to the editor, sir?" Arthur answered: "I don't think it would do much good. Dr. Stanley is the editor" (Baker Service).

The point of the above vignette is not that medical researchers falsify their results and, unless one is careful, one will be misled.[4] More likely, Arthur was having some fun at Stanley's expense (Stanley was a former attending at Pacific). He was using humor to pass a lesson on to his subordinates: the logic of your own experience determines the usefulness of the research of others.

Scientific evidence takes its meaning in the light of the current clinical situation and past clinical experience.

The passing on of clinical expertise also allows for a more collegial relation to develop than scientific evidence alone provides. It allows superordinates to induct subordinates into the secrets of the profession. Often attendings on rounds will ask subordinates to project a clinical plan of action, praise them for the formal correctness of their answers, and then point out how such plans are nevertheless inappropriate given the nature of the situation:

Mrs. Sharper was admitted complaining of abdominal pain. She had been operated on twice at another hospital in the area and to Arthur it was "obvious" that her problems were iatrogenic. He claimed that of the two surgeons who had operated on her earlier, the first is a "heavy-handed son-of-a-bitch," and the second is "untalented, but he married well." Then Arthur asked Christian what he thought should be done. Christian replied that he would like to run a series of tests to determine the extent of the damage and that then they should go in and make the necessary correction, revising the work of the other surgeons.

Arthur replied that under ideal conditions, Christian was right; but for this patient it would be unwise to revise the damage of the earlier surgeons. They should go in and relieve her difficulty and they should do that stat [immediately]. Arthur said that this should be done not because it was a life-threatening situation nor because it was an emergency, but because "Mrs. Sharper is a seventy-four-year-old woman and when you get old people in the hospital, put them on their backs in bed, start running IV tubes into them, and placing nasogastric tubes down them, they die. It never fails. The best thing to do with old people is to get them in and out of the hospital as quickly as possible."

To give evidence for this assertion, Arthur told the story of an experience that he had as an intern, one that had made "a damn strong impression on him, one that he'd never forget." The story went as follows: One of his first rotations was on

the service of a surgeon who did prostate operations for
wealthy patients at "a thousand a shot." Arthur claimed,
"Now, that's a lot of money but well worth it if your bladder
is obstructed." One of Arthur's first patients was an old man
needing a prostate operation done, but he also had com-
plicating problems that required extensive tests. And, as
Arthur related it, "That son-of-a-bitch died before we had a
chance to operate." Arthur learned the following lesson from
the experience which he passed on to the group: "While I
am as you know quite conservative about preoperative care
[*conservative* here means he requires a lot], for old people,
like this lady, just get them in and out as fast as possible before they die on you. Fart around and they'll die. I swear it.
It never fails" (Baker Service).

Mrs. Hooper, a patient on the Able Service, has a huge lump
in the groin area. Dr. White asked Paul what course of action
he would recommend if the lump turned out to be a sarcoma
[a malignant tumor of the muscle]. Paul answered that he
thought hip disarticulation [removal of leg at hip joint]
would be the operation of choice. White agreed that it would
be the operation of choice, but stated that he would not
recommend it in this case: "I don't think this lady could live
with a hip disarticulation. She's relatively obese and I don't
think that she would tolerate the procedure very well. She'd
be confined to a wheelchair the rest of her life. I've had
patients do remarkably well with hip disarticulation, but not
in this case. I think I'll just have to scoop it out as best I
can." He then added facetiously, "Maybe it's cat-scratch
fever. There's a big run on cat scratches these days."
"Unfortunately she doesn't have a cat," said Paul. "I know,"
answered White. "But I think we can get good results
scooping it out. I once had a patient with an invasive tumor
that I just kept scooping out. I was able to save his leg for ten
years that way," added Dr. Peters (Able Service).

Through such exchanges, attendings communicate to subordinates a number of messages. First, they pass on what considerations should lead one to modify conventional wisdom. Second,
they allow attendings to support a subordinate's performance
on one level while, on another level, they allow the attending to

change it. The attending's citation of lessons learned from his own clinical history indicates to subordinates how much they have left to learn. Third, these exchanges communicate a certain, albeit limited, sympathy that attendings have for the plight of their subordinates. In such exchanges one of the things that a superordinate is telling his subordinate is, "Look, we all learn the hard way. I did; you will."

> On Able Service, we entered Mrs. Grout's room, a patient with metastatic cancer. While in the hospital she was given penicillin for a secondary infection. Although she reported no known history of allergy and although there was nothing in the official record to indicate an allergy, she had an allergic reaction—hives, swollen face, and cold sores. Dr. Peters looked at her, told her she was doing much better, and left her room. Outside he said to Mark, "Sure is something, isn't it? Well, there's no way you could have known. I remember the first time I had a patient have an allergic reaction. Really made me respect the stuff. Made me very cautious about using it. I daresay that you'll think twice in the future before prescribing it." Mark said he would (Able Service).

This last message that the invocation of clinical expertise carried with it is rarely so forcefully stated as above. As a consequence, it is subject to much noise and distortion. Subordinates are often more aware of the critical rather than the supportive import of being overruled. Housestaff complain that they are not allowed to participate fully enough in decision making and that when an attending's actions are not supported by the facts, there is nothing they can do. In addition, the fact that arguments from personal clinical experience are compelling means that the attending is drawing on a store of private knowledge not available to subordinates. This reinforces in the mind of housestaff the stereotype of the arbitrary attending.

For their part, subordinates rely on scientific evidence to ground their decisions. This is quite natural since their stock of firsthand knowledge is so small. Sudnow (1967) notes the importance of "counting" in a hospital. Any individual counts events, that is, sees them as unique occurrences whose characteristics need attending to, until events of this type become for him a routine taken-for-granted part of the environment. In Sudnow's study, a veteran hospital worker is the one who has lost count of the deaths he has seen; a novice still counts and still catalogs—he still notices death. If Icheiser (1972) did not remind us that we are never so blind as when we are facing the "obvious," it might strike us as strange that persons die and others not notice. But a good working definition of a hospital is that place where death occurs and no one notices; or, more sharply, the place where others agree to notice death as a social fact only so far as it fits their particular purposes.

On a service there is great variation in the degree to which one notices death. Attendings and chief residents have stopped counting deaths; in all likelihood, junior medical students are so clinically uninitiated that they have not yet seen anyone die first-hand—they are ready to begin counting.

As far as it fits their particular purposes, for surgeons death ends their action. It is not unfair to recognize that there is a gladiator dimension to surgery and surgeons. Surgeons take up scalpel against disease; they resist with force its invasion on the body. When death comes, the struggle is ended. Little is said to the patient's family. Like prideful Achilles, the surgeon repairs to his tent and prepares for his next combat. Surgeons are not unaware of this dimension of their work. When one asks a surgeon why he chose to do this of all things medical, invariably in his reply he mentions the dramatic and decisive interventions that are the surgeon's. Surgeons report that they like being "where the action is" (Goffman 1961).

I mention this only to point out a relationship between task-structure and the moral and ethical division of labor. By and large, surgeons have not been contributors to the literature on death and dying. This is not by accident nor does it discredit the surgeon. Surgeons live within the bounds of a simple code; they view it as the task of others to articulate philosophies.

Exposure to clinical problems are the events that are significant enough for housestaff to keep track of, to count: a porta-

caval shunt [a connection of the main vein from the intestine to
the main vein from the lower body bypassing the liver], a hemi-
pelvectomy [removal of lower extremity and half the pelvis], for a
malignant schwannoma [a tumor of the nerve], a case of Zollin-
ger-Ellison syndrome [a tumor of the pancreas which causes the
stomach to secrete excess acid], or a gastroenterostomy [a connection of stomach to upper intestine], are big events in a houseofficer's development. Each new event provides impressions to
match against the clinical descriptions in the literature and each
exposure provides knowledge that can be used next time. Housestaff proceed by the book because they have not yet developed an
overly large and useful stock of knowledge. Yet following procedures—going by the book—has a virtue all its own: as long as
one has done this, one is protected from the damaging interpretations of failure. Better to blame bad luck than *hubris*:

> Mark had performed an esophagogastrectomy [removal of
> esophagus and stomach], on Mr. Warren. This was Mark's
> first, and he was being generally left alone by Arthur and
> Grant to manage the patient. (Mark's training has only six
> weeks left and the attendings are treating him very much as
> a colleague.) Mark has a special interest in Mr. Warren. His
> chief concern was whether his anastomosis would hold. He
> had taped a note to Mr. Warren's forehead forbidding any-
> one from moving the tube placed down Warren's nose, his
> fear being that the tube would rip the suture line. We were
> visiting Mr. Warren on morning rounds. Mark was pleased
> to see that there were no difficulties in the immediate post-
> operative period. Stan asked him when he intended to feed
> Mr. Warren. "Seven days," Mark answered. "You know
> Gray [an attending noted for his skill at this procedure] has
> them eating much faster than that. On the third day postop
> he already has them on clear liquids," Stan said. "I know,
> but let me try that and have it not work. They'd crucify me.
> Unh, unh! I want no part of that. Because, after all, this is
> only my hundred and first [with a heavy emphasis on *first*]
> esophagogastrectomy. I'm going to play it really straight"
> (Baker Service).

The guidelines in the scientific literature establish a standard of proper behavior for housestaff. The attending who does not follow these standards and cannot supply acceptable reasons for his deviations is often viewed by housestaff as "dogmatic" or "lacking in clinical judgment." The attending who does not follow these standards but can give acceptable reasons, that is, can extract generalizable lessons from his clinical experience, is respected by housestaff as a good teacher. Much more autocratic and much more eccentric behavior is tolerated without complaint in the second case than in the first.

The tension between clinical expertise and scientific evidence expresses the inequalities among ranks on a surgery service; it also expresses an even more basic tension of medical practice: the art of healing versus the science of medicine. Rule by clinical expertise emphasizes the "artful" dimensions of practice. The attending's claim of authority has an almost mystical quality: "Trust me, for I have seen." In the world of medicine, clinical acumen is a charismatic possession, a gift of grace; its exact nature is a mystery. On the other hand, rule by scientific evidence emphasizes the rational and technical dimensions of practice. The legitimation of scientific evidence is of the most routine nature; the exact nature of this authority is not mysterious but known to all. Operationally, these two types of legitimation are resources that actors in a scene possess to justify a course of action. Attendings possess both types of authority. In contrast, their subordinates have little science, less clinical expertise. As a consequence, attendings always have the unanswerable argument. Although an attending's authority is in some formal sense always legitimate, unless his authority is respected by virtue of both his clinical and scientific expertise, then his subordinates are likely to experience his leadership as interference, to avoid his control whenever possible, and to grouse to others about the attending's shortcomings.

Subordinates resent the attending's power to construct a binding definition of reality for good reason. One of those binding definitions that an attending makes is whether or not an individual should be allowed to progress through training. At-

tending rounds are an occasion for the attending to determine
through questioning the sophistication of a subordinate's reasoning, to observe whether a subordinate works hard enough to get
adequate results, to appraise if a subordinate has any personality
problems that prevent him from doing decent work, and to
judge in general whether the subordinate promises to be worth
the effort it takes to train a surgeon. This judgment is legitimated
on the basis of the clinical expertise an attending has developed
through his teaching experience. As with the invocation of clinical expertise in patient care, the subordinate has no remedies if
he finds himself in disagreement with clinical wisdom. If he is
asked to leave a training program, the subordinate cannot appeal
the decision, show how it was biased and the facts of the situation
misread, and then be reinstated. The dismissed subordinate
must find a place somewhere else or give up any hope of becoming a board-certified surgeon.[5] The fact that such decisions
are legitimated by clinical expertise means that they are both
unanswerable and unanalyzable—they are as mysterious as the
source of this authority. Not surprisingly, this is a major resentment and tension of housestaff before they enter the upper end of
the pyramid and are relatively secure:

> I really dislike the autocratic nature of surgery. Attendings
> piss you off and there's nothing you can do. And if you piss
> attendings off they can screw you. Some attendings are really
> vindictive. They have no concern for us at all (Resident).

> On Baker Service, Arthur had complained bitterly after
> rounds about the quality of work. Josh had felt the criticism
> was unfair and he complained to me: "Let me tell you some-
> thing: this is a pyramid program and in a few weeks these
> guys are going to sit down and decide who to keep for senior
> residents. And when you get kicked out of a program you
> don't move to Mass. General. You move laterally if you're
> lucky, really lucky, or you move downward. You make one
> public enemy like this bastard and he can ruin your career. I
> don't know what it's like for you in graduate school, but if
> you want to get through this training program you'd better be
> prepared to swallow a whole lot of shit." I assured him there

was some shit in graduate school and asked if there was any
way to disagree with an attending. "How can you? It doesn't
matter if you're right; they can still screw you. The only time
you could do anything is if you decided that you didn't want
to stay here and you really didn't care where you went next.
Then maybe you could hit back when they lash out at you.
But as it is now you have no choice but to take whatever they
dish out without being able to defend yourself. It doesn't
matter whether you're right or wrong or anything. You just
have to take it (Baker Service).

The fact that clinical judgment is the basis for evaluation
unsettles housestaff. They see decisions concerning patient
management that seem arbitrary and contrary to the demands of
science justified by clinical expertise; they are dressed-down for
quasi-normative errors which are mistakes only from the idiosyncratic perspective of an individual attending; and they see that
their interpretation of events is of little importance. Because of
this, they fear the possibility of being unfairly evaluated; and
because these evaluations are on such relatively unspecified
grounds, those dismissed may always claim they were unfairly
treated, the victims of a malevolent attending. The intensity of
these beliefs may blind us to another function of clinical expertise—that is, such expertise is also the basis of the toleration and
forgiveness of subordinate errors. The attending's judgment in
these cases does not alienate his subordinates but rather creates
strong allegiances and debts that subordinates must repay by a
higher standard of work in the future. What we are concerned
with at present is, given such a system of authority, how does the
attending construct a judgment of his subordinates? How do
ward rounds function as a competence quiz? This brings us to the
questioning process by which superordinates test subordinates.

The Questioning Process

To understand how attendings judge the performance of subordinates, it is necessary to examine how subordinates are questioned. To do so, we have to recall two considerations developed

above: (1) there are two different orders of failure: an account either sustains or subverts a normal definition of the situation; and (2) an attending by virtue of the preeminence of clinical expertise has the right to construct the binding interpretation of reality—an attending need not modify his claims about what is happening because of the counterclaims of housestaff. Given this, we may speak of how meanings about the quality of performance are negotiated, all the time recognizing that there are limits to the meaningfulness of calling these negotiations since an attending can break off discussion at any point.

Basically, we can describe the questioning process on rounds as an attempt to establish to what order subordinate performance belongs: is a subordinate failing to meet minimal role requirements and by such behavior making normative or quasi-normative breaches; or is he a reasonable and responsible subordinate whose only errors are the technical and judgmental errors of inexperience? The chief weapon that the attending uses to find out is the question. As Sacks's chain-rule for questions establishes (Churchill 1971), the proper etiquette for question-answer-question-answer sequences is, after the reply, the floor belongs to the questioner. Linguistic practice here subserves the needs of social rank. The superordinate can and does question subordinates until he receives an account that renders further questions unnecessary for his purposes. In a sense then, the attending's control of resources is extraordinary—not only can he construct a binding definition of reality, but there are no inherent limits which he must respect in questioning his subordinates.

Earlier I stated that the amount of monitoring is inversely related to an attending's evaluation of a subordinate. We must now go beyond this generalization and see how the judgment that performance is either acceptable or not is constructed on a day-to-day basis on rounds. When work is proceeding without incident and after subordinates have earned the trust of superordinates, there is not much monitoring of performance. There is a relaxed tone to decision making. Subordinates find it easier to tolerate the whims of superordinates, and superordinates find the gestures for independence of subordinates more acceptable:

On morning work rounds, we were in Mrs. Morrow's room.
Mark ordered that her subclavian line [an intravenous tube
from arm into large veins in neck] be discontinued. "I don't
think you want to do that, Mark," John said. "Why?" John:
"Yesterday on rounds, Grant [Mrs. Morrow's attending] said
he wanted it kept until she's eating a lot." Mark: "Okay.
Keep it in. I can't see what difference it makes either way."
As we left the room, Stan began talking to me. "I guess
you've noticed that when things are going well, our decisions
are not terribly important. Whether an IV is in for a day or
so longer, whether a patient is on clear or full liquids, it
doesn't matter much so long as they are getting better. But
when things are bad, and life is at stake, then these same
decisions are crucial" (Baker Service).

Surgeons do not like to disturb success any more than anyone
else. When there is little at stake for participants, routine and
minor encroachments of autonomy are easily tolerated. In fact,
as long as things go on smoothly, such little things tend to go
unnoticed by actors.

However, when work is not proceeding smoothly or when it is
early in a rotation and subordinates have not yet earned the trust
of attendings, rounds can be a very intense competence quiz with
a complete accounting for action demanded. After attendings
have sniffed around some by inspecting dressings and wounds
and by listening to lung fields and the like, questioning begins.
First, are questions of a general nature, such as "How is this
patient doing?" Equally general answers, such as "Fine," do not
suffice:

I'm sure you've heard me ask, "How's this patient?" and
heard someone answer "Fine." Well, I don't want impressions. I want the facts. If someone says a patient is fine—
especially if I don't trust them—I'll ask further: "What
are the blood counts?" Anyone can say a patient is fine, but
that doesn't tell you much about your patient (Attending).

Look—you've heard us say on rounds, "Don't give me impressions. I don't give a good goddamn how a patient looks. Give
me numbers" (Attending).

The subordinate who answers superordinate questions with vague responses is presumed to be covering his ignorance, while the subordinate who answers general questions with technically complete responses or who, in informing an attending of a change in a patient's condition, is as complete as possible wins an attending's trust:

> The intern who calls you up and says X has a fever does not inspire your trust; but the intern who calls and says X has a urinary tract infection is altogether different. He reports the symptoms, gives you his diagnosis, and tells you what he plans to do. I don't need housestaff to tell me my patients have fevers—any secretary can do that—good housestaff take a little more initiative (Attending).

The subordinate who requires further questioning has by this fact alone led an attending to question his competence and trustworthiness. The attending must spend a great effort on this subordinate just to get an accurate reading of the situation. Questions follow in rapid succession: What are the blood counts? What did the latest chest film show? When is the barium swallow scheduled? Such questions are an attempt to establish if a subordinate at least knows what is going on with a patient. If a subordinate knows the facts of a case, questioning can move on to questions of treatment; but if a subordinate does not know what is going on with a patient, then the reason for this must be established. Here, there is only one acceptable defense: "The lab has not completed the test yet." Any other excuse such as "It's not my patient" or "I was off last night" indicate to an attending that a subordinate is not putting forth minimal effort to meet the requirements of his role. When such excuses are offered, an attending often dresses-down his subordinate. When the subordinate offers no excuses, the subordinate may be spared the dressing-down, although the attending usually finds other indirect methods for communicating his displeasure. Common tactics are to ignore the offender—literally to act as if he were not there—or to be exaggeratedly formal. In either case, the superordinate steps up monitoring. This results in an attending finding more and more things not to his liking. It is this that is the deviance-amplifying effect of monitoring: the actual rate of unacceptable practice may not increase, but the number of discovered instances rises. A very similar thing may be going on in the current malpractice crisis. It seems very unlikely that the rise in suits reflects an actual rise in negligent practice. More likely, a heightened sensitivity on the part of the lay public to the possibility that bad results are the consequence of bad practice encourages the suit as a remedy. What the rise in suits may speak to is a weakening of the physician's charisma and the evolution of a more formally contractual physician-patient relationship. There is a second striking parallel to this stepped-up monitoring of physicians: complaints about fee-seeking attorneys are similar to those housestaff make of attendings.

Once a subordinate establishes that he knows the facts of a case, questioning moves on to the next level, treatment. Here the subordinate must demonstrate that he knows what medications the patient is receiving and for what indications. A subordinate's ignorance is again evidence for an attending that the subordinate is not meeting the minimal requirements of his role. From this, it is not a great distance that an attending must travel logically to conclude that errors do not result from inexperience but from lack of concern for the norms and quasi-norms of good clinical practice. The subordinate who is found wanting here is in trouble in at least the short run and perhaps the long. Subordinates for their part feel that there are good reasons to explain why they might not know what is going on in any particular patient. They are angered by the attending's refusal to give these accounts a hearing. They complain that attendings are insensitive to physical demands placed on them:

> Carl was upset about Thelma Halsted's death. He blamed
> himself for missing some of the physical signs of cardiogenic
> shock [shock from heart failure], and then he blamed the
> conditions under which he was expected to work: "You can't
> really do this job unless you get some rest. I stress rest
> because we're so tired we're not people, we're robots. You'd

be surprised how depressed cerebral function is when you're
really tired. And when you're here everyday thinking about
surgical problems, you don't notice other things. Look—I
know all the signs of heart failure. Christ, she was frothing at
the mouth. I'm sure she had pulmonary edema [filling of
lungs with fluid]. I know the signs, but they're not in the
front of my mind, you know, because I'm thinking about
pararectal abscesses [abscess adjacent to rectum], or wound
infections, and you don't always put together what is under
your nose. Today's thing, that's our fault. Last night she
should have had an emergency heart consultation, but it was
so late, we were so tired, we thought that it could wait until
morning" (Able Service).

Or subordinates claim that attendings' expectations are unrealistic and, if taken seriously, would require them to be in two
places at the same time:

Ernest and Josh were discussing the dressing-down Josh had
just received from Arthur and Grant. Josh repeated to
Ernest, who had missed rounds, a comment of Grant's that
attending rounds were for teaching but today so much
routine work had to be done, such as dressing changes, that
rounds had been a waste of everybody's time. Ernest told
Josh that this was probably the thing that pissed Arthur and
Grant off the most. Josh asked how the ward work could be
done if Arthur demanded that everybody be in the operating
room on surgery days. Josh mentioned that this morning they
had been down on the ward doing the scut only to get paged
so that they "could stand around and watch Arthur." Ernest
answered that as Josh knew it was Arthur's philosophy that
all housestaff be in the OR on surgery days, that even if
housestaff weren't actually doing the case they could learn
from watching Arthur. Ernest added that he thought
Arthur was right as far as that was concerned. Josh replied:
"Okay, then he shouldn't be pissed off if the work isn't
always done or if it was screwed up by some inexperienced
junior student." Ernest answered: "That's just the point.
Arthur assumed that since you weren't in the OR all day,
you were here doing the ward work. Look, you finished the

first case at 10:00 A.M. and you were in the second one
only from 11:30 to 1:00. So when the ward work wasn't
done, Arthur thought you were just goofing off" (Baker
Service).

Attendings accept no excuses when they decide that a subordinate shows them he has not been working hard enough to
meet minimal role requirements, to master the fundamentals
of patient care. Such subordinates are seen as simply not working hard enough, carefully enough, or seriously enough and
they are embarrassing the standards of patient care. Such
embarrassment is not gladly suffered by attendings; in fact, it
is not even tolerated. Yet it remains true that attendings spot
such lapses through a random check of behavior and then
generalize from it that an intern who does not even do this
must not be doing other things as well. This method of discovery keeps alive in subordinates the fear that a random and
unrepresentative event will cause them to be stigmatized. What
an attending sees and what he might see but does not notice is
the bedrock phenomena from which housestaff construct the
categories "good and bad luck." There are as a rule a number
of ways in which luck is not with the subordinate, and we have
outlined some of these above. There are also a number of ways
in which good fortune is with the subordinate, the ways in
work is organized to prevent an attending from noticing poor
performance. First, the subordinate rotates through a number
of services; this lessens the probability of substandard work
being spotted since each attending observes him for only a
short period (usually only eight weeks). Second, the corporate
nature of the service responsibility often means that those who
know what is going on may rescue those that do not. There is
the "filling in" that occurs during work rounds; and there is
the attending's practice of asking questions generally to the
group rather than directly to individuals.

The first step of attending rounds, the first order of questions, establishes if subordinates are "on top of a situation,"
that is, if their organization of effort is meeting the basic

expectations of their superiors. The first level of questions discriminates subordinates into the worthy and the unworthy. Superordinates then move on to questions about the theoretical adequacy of the work done. This second level of questions rank-orders those who are considered worthy. At the second level of questioning, the attending shifts the focus from "what" to "why." He asks a subordinate to explain the reasons why he has done what he has done and what he hopes to effect by the course of his action. To an attending the subordinate's answer indicates his sophistication at medical reasoning. If the subordinate fails utterly, he may find himself back at the first-order questions. If the subordinate errs but indicates a grasp of the situation, the attending leads him through a reasoning exercise. Checks on reasoning may be made retrospectively or prospectively. Prospective checks are safest for attendings, patients, and housestaff. The reasoning exercises that attendings lead housestaff and students through is the way clinical expertise is passed on. This way of learning to make a diagnosis is one of the principal activities of clinical-medical education. For students and housestaff the process is the same: the examination of evidence and then a dialogue with the attending. In the episode below there are two such reasoning exercises: one of Arthur with Larry and one with Tom. Especially noteworthy is the quick and sarcastic way Larry is dismissed when he demonstrates that he does not know what is going on, as against the enthusiastic and almost collegial way Arthur expands Tom's suggestion:

We were in X ray. Arthur asked Tom, the senior student, "Do we have any interesting pictures for today?" "Just the consult from Gen Med." Arthur turned to a junior student: "Okay, Larry, what does this lesion suggest to you as your diagnosis?" "Ulcerative colitis?" Larry asked more than he answered. "Absolutely not. Try again." Larry suggests something weird. Arthur answers him: "I've only seen three cases of that in all my clinical experience! C'mon, think, will you! What did he get close to—a plane, and a propeller sliced off that portion of his colon? It's a tumor—I'm sure it's a cancer." Mark added: "On the diagnosis, you'd have to list it as

about eight and a half of the first ten possibilities." Arthur:
"Nine and a half. Okay, Tom, what should we do about it?
[A pause] Tom?" "I'm here. I was just thinking. I guess a left
colectomy or a total colectomy." Arthur: "This is a young
man. He's only thirty-eight. I think we should go for broke
and try to cure him. A total colectomy [total removal of colon
and rectum] and an ileostomy [an externalization of the lower
intestine]. We can cut it away and he can be cured and live
forty more years. Why be half-assed and risk recurrence?
This man's young. Is there any history of cancer in his
family?" Mark: "I don't believe so." "Then there is an eight
percent recurrence rate. That's pretty high, but it is much
higher with a history. This guy is only thirty-eight. It's really
unusual for cancer to appear in such a young guy—it's a real
tragedy. [To Grant] What a fascinating lesion! Let's put it
on the tumor clinic for Friday. It's tremendously unfortunate
for the patient, but it really is an interesting case. Poor
bastard" (Baker Service).

Moreover, this exchange also suggests an interesting ambivalence
of medical problems: namely, what is most exciting and interesting is often most tragic. By such interchanges clinical judgment is
formed. The subordinate suggests and the attending corrects. A
persistent and recurring problem then is the attending who corrects but neglects to give his reasons. Housestaff feel that this is
an abuse of rank.

There are several things to consider about controls at the
second level, or what I have called the "why?" level of questioning. First, mistakes at this level are assumed to be more correctable than mistakes at the first level. Second, the knowledge that
a subordinate's reasoning is flawed is apt to build slower than
first-level mistakes. Reasoning mistakes are seen as reflecting the
current state of a subordinate's art; it is harder for attendings to
see such mistakes as part of a pattern. Third, mistakes at the
second level do not engage as much of the subordinate's self in
the evaluation as mistakes at the first level. First-level mistakes
imply to attendings some sort of character defect. Second-level
mistakes imply only a lack of exposure to the proper material.

The Horror Story

As we have described them, the social controls established by
attending rounds are both flexible and harsh. They are harsh in
that the minimum standards set for acceptable work are quite
high and there are no acceptable excuses for not meeting these
standards. They are flexible in that once an individual has
demonstrated an ability and a willingness to meet these minimal,
albeit difficult, demands of the job, there are acceptable excuses
for error and mistakes. These mishaps become a routine part of
the environment and serve to reinforce a training definition of the
situation. We have described how the preeminence of clinical
expertise allows an attending to construct a binding interpretation of reality and how this power creates tensions among subordinates and between superordinates and subordinates. Now we
turn to one feature of social life among surgeons that tends to
dissipate everyday tensions to some degree—the horror story.

Horror stories, grotesque catalogs of all the things that can go
wrong in treating patients, abound in the hospital. From these
stories, we should not infer that hospitals deliver slipshod care;
rather, these stories should be seen as moral parables, an element
of the oral culture of medicine that remind all that healing is a
difficult business that must always be done with care. Evidence
that some horror stories may be apocryphal is the following: I
have heard different physicians-in-training in different types of
hospitals in different geographic regions repeat the same horror
stories. These stories have the quality of "just-so" tales: the
action is set in the past, exactly when no one can recall, and the
characters are persons whose names cannot be recalled. Horror
stories are told in two different ways. An attending may in the
course of events pass a story on to a subordinate. Attendings tell
three types of story. First is the cautionary parable:

> On attending rounds on Able Service, Peters asks: "What was
> this patient admitted with?" Carl answers: "Gastrointestinal
> bleeding in the emergency room." "And what did you do?"
> "Applied nasogastric suction and started an IV." Peters then

asks: "And where did these ministrations take place? In the ER?" "On the floor." "Then you admitted the patient?" Carl: "Why, yes, of course." Peters explains: "Well, that's very important and shouldn't be taken for granted. Last month, a friend of one of the staff went to the ER with gastrointestinal bleeding and was sent home. He bled to death. It's very important to remember to admit. What I'm doing is keeping the lesson alive" (Able Service).

Of all horror stories, there are more variants of this than any other I heard. In some versions, the "friend of the staff" is a "visiting dignitary to the Pacific community." When housestaff exchange the story among themselves, they invariably add that the resident who treated the patient was dismissed the next morning. The story drives home in a very concise way the need for caution, care, and completeness. It allows an attending to communicate this by sharing a bit of hospital lore with his subordinate rather than by directly criticizing performance.

A second type of horror story that attendings exchange with subordinates communicates the shared difficulties that they face as surgeons:

Mark joined the Able Service late on rounds. As we left a patient's room, White addressed him: "I hear you had some problems up there [the operating room]." "Yeah. I couldn't get the damn wound to stop oozing. I was getting pretty aggravated. I thought that the anesthesiologists might have given too much heparin [an anticoagulant]. But they had written down one unit so I couldn't blame them." White continued: "I figured something like that was happening when you weren't down here. When I left you were ready to sew her up. It is possible that the anesthesiologists gave too much heparin. I once had a patient die that way. I once ordered three units of heparin and the patient was mistakenly given three ten-unit doses. So, instead of three thousand units, he had thirty thousand units. We achieved some hemostasis [stopping bleeding], but the patient died soon after." Mark pointed out that "they don't keep those bottles in the OR any more." "Yes, I know. I made a real big stink downstairs and demanded that they all be removed" (Able Service).

Such stories cataloging how the good work of surgeons at Pacific is frustrated by others are quite common. Radiologists and anesthesiologists are favorite targets, as are specialists in internal medicine. The tales told about this latter group record as a rule how their excessive caution and indecision prevent surgeons from coming to the aid of patients until it is too late. Arthur is able to recall numerous occasions when he was asked to consult on patients in such advanced stages of disease that they were dead within forty-eight hours. Another favorite source of such stories are the surgeons at less prestigious hospitals who refer their difficult problems to Pacific. The surgeons at Pacific even have contemptuous terms for such physicians and their patients: the physicians are LMDs (local medical doctors) and their patients are "suburban specials." Mumford (1970) notes the same labeling phenomenon among the housestaff in the elite hospital she studied. The surgeons at Pacific tell stories of how they have received patients in the emergency room with no more information than "Pacific Hospital, Intensive Care" pinned to their nightshirts. The dumps of others become horror stories:

At one point on rounds, we stopped to discuss a patient referred from a hospital in a predominantly Jewish suburb. Arthur spoke: "That's one place that has killed more Jews than Eichmann. I can think of any number of atrocities committed there. Mr. Silver we salvaged through no fault of theirs. This one guy really pisses me off. He's been at at least two lectures where I've discussed the problem he sent us today and what does he do? An idiot stunt like taking out the appendix. That's like cutting down a tree to stop a forest fire. I can think of a few other patients he has killed. On one man, he removed most of the small bowel." "Jesus!" One student murmured. Arthur replied: "Yeah, that fellow met Jesus all right!" Rounds then continued (Baker Service).

Such stories circulate quite frequently. They are a way for surgeons to express open disapproval of behavior that they cannot control. They are also, in an oblique way, defensive. The horror stories within the surgery department at Pacific occur for all to see; informing others of the disasters that happen elsewhere is a way for surgeons to claim: "What you see here may not be perfect, but it pales in comparison to what goes on elsewhere."

There is a third type of horror story that attendings tell their subordinates. This involves telling jokes on themselves. Between operations, in time-out periods, attendings recount the great adventures of their training. Such stories routinely recount their troubles with those surgeons who were their attendings. They indicate that attendings understand that mishaps are a normal part of training; that, indeed, such things have happened to them; and that they survived them. Moreover, the more off-color of these stories involve some conflict between duty and fun, usually symbolized by sex and alcohol. The values of a male culture are celebrated in locker-room language. Even in the tamest of such stories, the value of grace under pressure, professional cool, is upheld:

> Toward the end of rounds, Arthur asked if anyone knew which island Hippocrates was from. When no one could answer, he turned to Grant and said: "Grant, it looks like you and I are the only two educated people on this service. Don't they teach you people any history of medicine?" Ernest answered that in his first year there were two noncredit lectures but he had been too busy to go. Grant stated that the history of medicine used to be studied if only to know the eponyms: "For instance, if you call something the 'Ernest syndrome,' the natural question is, 'Who is Ernest?'" Everyone laughed and Brian stepped forward: "We're laughing because we have discovered the 'Ernest syndrome.'" "Oh? What's that?" asked Arthur. "It's a patient with a left radical mastectomy who has a tattoo on the right contralateral thigh. It's named for Mrs. Fogg," answered Brian. Arthur laughed and added that during his training residents were given eponyms by attendings for stupid things that they had done: "For example, the Hammersmith phenomenon occurs when the resident cuts the attending's hand while removing the specimen. I remember when I got my eponym. I was doing my first total colectomy [total removal of colon and

rectum], with Dr. Cranz and he did it a little differently
than we do now. He clipped off the specimen with hemostats
[a small clamp]; he didn't tie it off the way we do now. Anyway, the specimen was out and I was bored sitting there
holding an idiot stick [a retractor] and the two other residents were removing hemostats from the specimen. They left
two on so I thought I'd be helpful and I reached up and
removed the hemostats just as the hemostat was perfectly
above the open wound and this liquid feces comes pouring
out. I thought to myself I'd better see when the first train
leaves for home. But Cranz didn't bat an eye. He just said,
'My, this is an unexpected development!' So he immediately
gets the sucker going to clean the wound. And he irrigated
the wound with a couple buckets of saline, and the operation
went on as if nothing had happened. The patient didn't bat
an eyelash recovering, and Dr. Cranz didn't say anything to
me until about a week after the patient left, when he said,
'You know, Arthur, that patient whom you performed the
intraperitoneal fecal lavage [an accidental washing of the
abdominal cavity with feces] on did very well.' So an intraperitoneal fecal lavage became known as the Arthur phenomenon" (Baker Service).

Needless to say, attendings do not tell such stories about themselves at the same time that they are dressing-down subordinates
for poor performance. Routinely, such stories are circulated after
an attending has "talked to" a subordinate and after the message has had some time to sink in. For the attending, telling a
horror story on himself is in a sense an attempt to reintegrate
both himself and his subordinates into a work group by matching
the humiliation he has forced on housestaff with some he willingly takes on himself. The second type of horror story on the
folly of others also has an integrative dimension since it includes
the auditor in the group of trusted people. As a general rule,
horror stories help transform outsiders into insiders by passing on
to them the secrets of the profession.

Horror stories are also told among subordinates themselves.
Here again the stories seem to fit one of three categories: (1)
directed against self, (2) directed against attendings, and (3)
directed against workers in the hospital. There are some routine

differences among the horror stories that attendings tell and the ones subordinates tell among themselves. First, the others that subordinates direct their stories against are usually lower-status workers in the hospital. Attendings never bother to tell stories about ancillary personnel. This reflects a difference between housestaff and attendings in whom they deal closely with: the point of the stories remains the same—those whom one relies on the most closely can destroy good work:

> On Able Service, a junior student told the following story that he had heard: A nurse's aide was assigned to watch a woman on a respirator. A patient at the other end of the hall had a cardiac arrest. The aide left the room to see what the commotion was about. The patient on the respirator turned her head and the tube kinked. By the time the nurse's aide returned, the cardiac monitor indicated a stopped heart. The patient was resuscitated but a vegetable. Three days later she died. The nurse's aide went undisciplined (Able Service).

> Today, Mr. Harmon claimed that he had been hurt by an X-ray technician in the ER and he asked for a shot of painkiller. As we left the room, Bill, the senior student, remarked that that technician had a reputation for being tough on patients. Bill said that when he was on a Gen Med rotation, a drunken man came in with a blow to the head. A subclavian line was inserted and X rays were ordered. At first, the technician refused to take the X rays. Then, when forced to, he treated the patient so roughly that he pulled out the subclavian and cracked the patient's ribs (Able Service).

A second difference between attending and housestaff horror stories concerns the way in which the stories are told. Subordinates circulate horror stories in a much more ritualized manner than do attendings. Two elements of story-telling practice are noteworthy. The stories themselves involve the sharing of various "firsts"—the first cutdown [entering a vein through an incision], the first proctoscopy [examination of rectum through a tube inserted into anus], the first intensive diagnostic study, and so on. These stories involve a catalog of all the things that can go wrong

on the most routine procedure. In a sly way, these stories express
an appreciation of and a sympathy for patients who provided
early clinical experience:

> Stuart was telling us about his first intensive diagnostic study.
> He had noticed an abnormally low blood chemistry reading on
> a preadmission test. He showed the reading to the resident.
> For the next hour, he and the resident marched in and out of
> the patient's room asking about all sorts of strange diseases
> and symptoms. The patient became visibly nervous. Another
> blood test was given and the readings came back normal.
> Something had gone wrong in the computer (Able Service).

> We were talking outside the area where proctoscopies were
> done. Mark was telling us a story a friend had told him about
> his first proctoscopy. "He couldn't understand it. He couldn't
> get the proctoscope in at all. So he looks down and sees what
> he's done to this woman and without turning a hair he says,
> 'Well, that one is just perfect—great. Now hold on a few
> seconds longer while we get a look at the other opening down
> there'" (Able Service).

> Josh was retelling a story from his cardiac rotation: "It was
> the first time I was going to change a battery on a pace-
> maker. There was just me and this medical student in the OR
> and the patient had a cardiac arrest right after I put in the
> local anesthetic. I spent an hour and a half working on the
> guy while the anesthesiologist picked his nose. I was sure I
> was going to be out on my ass" (Baker Service).

Next, stories proceed in a one-up fashion and become increas-
ingly more grotesque and macabre. Such story telling is an
anteing-up of clinical credentials on the part of housestaff. Having a ready stock of stories serves notice that one has been around
and knows what is going on.

The majority of stories that subordinates tell among themselves
are directed against themselves. These stories serve a number of
functions. First, like laughter, they relieve anxiety at the same
time that they express it. This anxiety is usually over the fit
between the person and the healer role. The highly ritualized

form of the stories, especially the emphasis on inexperience, makes this anxiety all the more clear. Horror stories allow participants to communicate in a backhand way their awe at the tasks before them, their reverence for sound clinical judgment and experience, their apprehensions about the levels of their skills, and the secret knowledge that one learns from misadventure. Horror stories allow surgeons to comment on how ill the title "doctor" sometimes clothes the wearer. Second, horror stories allow guilt to be communicated and shared. These tales act to mitigate the strong norms of the role that prohibit physicians from expressing their feelings. Daniels (1961) presents a good discussion of how these norms are communicated in training. Third, horror stories are cautionary parables—they instruct the beginner that pride goeth before a fall.

Horror stories, then, are a recurring feature of behavior which helps mitigate the tensions of surgical training. By circulating secret knowledge such stories help recreate a sense of group after dressing-downs. As a rule, superordinates tell such stories for their heuristic value, but they also serve as a bit of comedy that relaxes tensions. Subordinates use these stories to establish their credentials as members of the group of surgeons. A repertoire of tales indicates a depth of experience. At the same time, horror stories allow access to affective dimensions of the self that normal fulfillment of the role denies. As such, they are a social control of the harsher aspects of ward rounds.

four

The
Legitimation
of Attending
Authority

We have so far seen how failure is managed at the level of the work group. We have discussed the types of accounts that are given when deaths and complications occur, seen how these accounts are distributed throughout the division of labor, and shown how everyday routine surveillance acts as a means for superordinates to prevent and/or minimize failure and evaluate subordinate performance. Two features of this system of social control are noteworthy. First, knowledge of everyday performance is limited to members of the work group. Other colleagues do not observe each other's work and what information they do receive is systematically biased hearsay. That is to say, attendings, as well as housestaff, are most likely to grouse among themselves and spread information in those cases where they feel that the objective fact of a death or complication reflects unfairly on their performance.[1] The segregation of everyday controls and the great range of expressive behavior that attendings are allowed in applying them permits us to characterize such controls as private or backstage performances (Goffman 1961).[2] Second, the power of attendings in the system of everyday controls is truly remarkable. They alone decide if mistakes are forgivable or not, if subordinates are trustworthy or not. The binding understandings of failure forged at the everyday level are the attending's. His tolerance of technical and judgmental errors creates loyalty among subordinates and encourages greater efforts from them in the future to repay the obligation incurred by the attending's forgiveness. The swift and harsh dressing-downs that follow normative and quasi-normative errors define the boundaries within which forgiveness is permissible. Intolerance here creates rage and anger among subordinates and weakens ties to superordinates.

These two features of everyday controls—their privacy and the
extent of the attending's authority—arrest our attention, first for
their everyday operation and short-run consequences and second,
and even more important, because they seem to indicate that the
system of social control and socialization rests on an internal
contradiction. On the one hand, one overarching norm governs
the evaluation of performance, the rule of "no surprises"; full
and complete disclosures are demanded of subordinates. Yet, on
the other hand, superordinates are at an everyday level free of this
constraint. The privilege of their rank is that they need not
provide subordinates with any explanations for their actions. This
freedom from the constraint of full and complete disclosure is
what Weber defines as authority. Simply stated, this is the attending's power to give orders and expect that they will be carried
out. Earlier we have seen what beliefs attendings invoke to legitimate their treatment of subordinates, that is, to justify their use
of authority. What we have not yet explained is how attendings
maintain this considerable authority. This is not an unimportant
question, for authority does not just exist; its holders must take
great pains to maintain it against persons and events that challenge it.

In this chapter we shall explore the ways attendings dramatize
their claims to authority and hence maintain it. Such dramatizations are important for a number of reasons. To begin with,
they help explain the stability of attending authority. This stability should not be taken for granted, because when deaths and
complications occur the primary responsibility is the attending's.
Failure contradicts the attending's claim to powers beyond his
housestaff in a public and undeniable fashion. Furthermore,
these dramatizations explain what factors limit superordinate
authority and allow subordinates to accept it despite its occasional arbitrariness. Also, by displaying what norms attendings
must satisfy in order to maintain their legitimacy, they show how
attendings meet the requirements of full and open disclosure
that they demand of subordinates. Such dramatizations remind
everyone that attendings remain accountable for their actions and
go a long way toward resolving the contradiction between what

attendings require of their housestaff and what they require of themselves.

The attending's claims of authority rest first and foremost on external symbols independent of his day-to-day performance. These are his training, his experience, and his research contributions; however, such reputational assets would mean little if not reaffirmed by day-to-day performance. Therefore, attendings must both explain their failures—that is, they must neutralize or divest failures of their negative meanings—and they must also make their successes highly visible. The privilege of the attending's rank is not that he is free from accountability but rather that the forum in which his accounts for failure are demanded, given, and accepted is much more formalized, ritualized, and polite than the forum he provides his houseofficers and, further, he is provided a special forum to celebrate his successes. These two forums are the Mortality and the Morbidity Conference and Grand Rounds, respectively. Below we shall analyze both as occasions which attendings use to legitimate their claims to authority. In so doing, we shall see how paradoxically the harshness underlying the system of social control is at the same time mitigated and reinforced.

Varieties of Normal Action

In chapter 1 I stated that the presumption of success, which is the only warrant for subjecting a patient to the risk and trauma of an operation, makes surgeons more accountable than other physicians for failure. I claimed that the surgeon's craft and his beliefs about it make surgeons sensitive to what failure implies about their skill and judgment. In chapters 2 and 3 I examined how attendings held housestaff accountable for their actions. I am now in a position to demonstrate how attendings transform the private troubles housestaff create for them into public issues in the Mortality and Morbidity Conference and Grand Rounds. Through these conferences attendings justify their claims to authority by public displays of virtuosity to the entire collegium of subordinates and superordinates. The accounting of attending surgeons is not a backstage activity but a very carefully staged presentation of self. Subordinate accounting is always a test of competence; superordinate accounting is always a display of confidence.

As with all social accounts, those offered in the Mortality and Morbidity Conference and Grand Rounds attempt to align discrepant outcomes and expectations. The possible relations among any actions, expectations, and outcomes can be simply conceptualized. To any action we attach either positive or negative expectations; the action therefore either achieves or fails to achieve its purposes. Merely for theoretic convenience are we assuming that action in everyday life shares definitive endings with dramatic action. Exactly when the curtain drops and the scene ends is itself often an issue in everyday life. People express their awareness of this by employing the following tactics to align discrepant expectations and outcomes: they attempt to suspend judgment and continue. They argue that the evidence is incomplete or that all the bugs in a plan are being worked out or, most boldly, that success has already occurred but is not yet visible. A good examination of this delaying tactic is found in Halberstam (1972). Surgery, however, does not afford the same opportunities as the Vietnam War for using this technique. The time horizon for determining outcomes is restricted in surgery. This is one of the features of the task-structure that makes surgeons so accountable. So, aware of the conceptual shortcomings involved, we can, nevertheless, combine these two dimensions of action to form a fourfold table that captures the possible relations among expectations and actions.

Action occurs in all cells, and groups evolve shared and patterned ways for treating such events. The more strained the fit of expectations and outcomes, the more shared and patterned the ways of treating them. The confusion and anxiety that occur when things turn out other than the way we have planned need resolution. In such cases more elaborate structures evolve for explaining the failure of our calculations than is the case when events emerge as planned. In this table, cells 1 (expected success) and 4 (expected failure) represent no-confusion events. Expectations and outcomes are congruent. No elaborated ground rules are needed for actors to explain events. Relations are relaxed and there is great variation in interpersonal styles.

Varieties of Normal Action

	Expectations	
	+	−
Outcomes +	**1** Expected Success	**2** Unexpected Success
−	**3** Unexpected Failure	**4** Expected Failure

Cells 2 and 3 are those in which more elaborate social accounting is necessary. These are confusing events. When an action turns out other than as planned it damns nothing so much as the power to diagnose a situation. Not surprisingly, the ability to diagnose a situation is something about which a physician cannot afford confusion. In the accounts offered to end this confusion, relations are formal and there is little variation in interpersonal styles. Cell 2 is unexpected success; accounting for it occurs in Grand Rounds. Cell 3 is unexpected failure; accounting for it occurs in the Mortality and Morbidity Conference, as well as at the everyday level that we described in chapters 2 and 3. As we shall see, the accounts offered in these two conferences differ substantially from those offered in the everyday face-to-face interaction among subordinate and superordinate.

No-Confusion Situations

Cell 1: Expected Success

In cell 1, where both expectations and outcomes are positive, we have routine, unquestioned successful action. In surgery as in everyday life, people do not ordinarily stop to question this action or challenge those persons who achieve results.[3] Given the didactic component of clinical training, it is not entirely accurate to state that attendings do not ask questions about routine and ordinary successes. They do. However, they need not ask these questions of their housestaff or of themselves. Routine success, the happily removed appendix or the artfully repaired hernia, threatens neither a houseofficer's nor an attending's credibility. On the contrary, such success anchors their claims of expertise in the empirical world and makes them substantial. However, such success may create problems for the medical student. Since routine success does not compel the attending to exert time and energy either keeping his subordinates in line or reexamining his own decisions, he has more time for testing his student's knowledge. Where the intern or resident is asked: "What went wrong?" "How did this happen?", the student is asked: "Why did this work?" "Why did we choose this course of action rather than some other?" Routinely such questioning is not very intense. The student serves as a convenient foil for the attending. Since this rotation is the student's first exposure to surgery, attendings do not always expect correct answers to such questions. Attendings use such questioning to expose and to impress on students their ignorance, to demonstrate the intellectual rigor needed for the surgical management of disease, and to illustrate some general principles of surgery.[4] Thus, even though routine and expected success may make an occasional student uncomfortable, it does not create confusion about what is going on. Colleagues do not take excessive notice when one simply meets the expectations of others. Only the most professionally infantile, the students, are invited to speculate about why success occurred. There is a parallel here to parents who ask children how simple objects work in order to demonstrate some simple causal relationships. Those initiated into a social world no longer wonder how such things work. They take them for granted. Action that falls in cell 1 ratifies the tacit assumptions on which surgery rests. It is not a topic for social accounting; rather, it is the background from which accountable events emerge.

Cell 4: Expected Failure

Cell 4, in which expectations and outcomes are negative, contains cases for which no elaborate social accounting is necessary. Patients who are hopelessly ill with terminal diseases fall into this category. What happens to these patients, although tragic, could not have been otherwise. According to Fox (1974), attitudes toward the discussion of the practical, existential, and ethical issues surrounding the care of the dying patient have changed considerably in medical schools over the last twenty years. What was formerly dismissed as merely philosophical is now openly discussed. In surgery, as in other areas of medicine, there is a concern for the humane treatment of dying patients. This en-larged discussion indicates a greater sensitivity on the part of medical educators to the fact that expected failure can be a trial on the personal and individual level at the same time that it is a normal event in a professional life. With the increased healing power of modern medicine there has arisen the need to make more explicit the individual strategies for handling the question, How do I recognize when a situation is hopeless and then what do I do? Confusion exists in this situation, to be sure, but this confusion is of a different order than that of cells 2 and 3, where expectations and outcomes are discrepant. The confusion that surrounds the hopeless cases of cell 4 is existential and individual. In cells 2 and 3, confusion is social and scientific. The difference is this: in cell 4, the physician must account for why an individual patient developed an untreatable cancer that both he and the patient would have preferred not to occur. In cell 2, he must account for how he salvaged an incurable. In cell 3 he must account for how he lost a curable. There is here a question of

responsibility. Cells 2 and 3 clearly raise questions of professional
responsibility. Cell 4 is at the boundary between individual and
human responsibility and professional responsibility. To help
their subordinates deal with the problems raised by the hopeless
cases of cell 4, attendings pass on to housestaff and students their
beliefs about when and how a patient should be allowed to die:

> We reached Mr. Starvos's room on rounds. We paused a long
> time before his door. Nothing was said. Everyone looked at
> the ceiling or down at the floor. Eye contact among people
> was not established. Finally Arthur said: "Goddammit." It
> was the group's signal to enter the room. Mr. Starvos com-
> plained of pain. He was alert and lucid. We left quickly.
> Arthur spoke: "He's too damned alert—that's all there is to
> it. Look, I'm not one to give up on patients but we have to
> realize that there comes a time when we can do nothing more
> for a patient and we should no longer support life but the let
> the patient die comfortably with as much dignity as pos-
> sible. In all honesty I think we have to admit we've reached
> that point with Mr. Starvos. He's too alert for that much
> pain. He shouldn't be that awake. Let's begin to give him
> Librium and morphine. Yeah—Librium and MS [mor-
> phine]—that should make him more comfortable. Mark, first
> talk to his wife. Make sure that his will is in order, all his
> bank accounts are square, and the property straight away.
> Then begin the Librium and MS. He's too alert. He needs
> sedation. Also, are they Catholic or Greek Orthodox? His
> wife was asking about a priest—I think it's time to tell her to
> bring him in. We can't do any more for him." The group
> saw one more patient on rounds and then Arthur mentioned
> Starvos again: "Look, there comes a time when you have to
> acknowledge your limits and make the patient as comfortable
> as possible. I think we can discontinue monitoring his vital
> signs at night. There's no reason to wake him up in the
> middle of the night to take his temperature, pulse, blood
> pressure, and all that other bullshit. Let's close the door,
> leave him with his family, and let him die with some dignity,
> as a man instead of a patient with a glass tube up his ass.
> We've done what we can. Let him die, poor man" (Baker
> Service).

On rounds, Arthur was discussing proper care of the dying patient. "You can't offer these patients shit but you have to go in there and perform a laying-on of hands, so to speak. You can't abandon them." The service had just visited a consult on the medical service and Arthur had decided that the patient's cancer was too advanced to warrant an operation. He continued: "That patient is terminal. Let's send her home with morphine and Librium and let her be with her family. If it was your mother, would you want her in the hospital? Remember that Chinaman they wanted us to operate on last week? He died forty-eight hours later. Christ, you could look at him and see that he was half dead—the medicine people said, 'No, it's because he's Chinese and they all look like that.' They'd be hanging IV's into their patients all the way to the morgue if we'd let them" (Baker Service).

There are, of course, grave differences of opinion on when it is the "proper time" to allow a patient to die with dignity. Surgeons are not known for throwing in the towel quickly. Nurses and physicians in other specialities are often critical of what they consider needless surgery, claiming that it extends suffering rather than life. Moreover, as a rule, subordinates are quicker than superordinates to decide that a patient is beyond help, a fact which is possibly more a comment on their control of treatment and their investment in its correctness than in their personal philosophies. But this is all quite beside the point: when it is expected, death threatens neither the professional self of the subordinate nor of his superior. One of the hard lessons that one must learn in surgery, as in all branches of medicine, is that there are times when nothing more remains to be done. Again, colleagues do not need to account when the unsalvageable are not salvaged. Action that falls into cell 4, like that which falls into cell 1, ratifies the tacit assumptions that make action in a scene possible, although these assumptions are of a different order. Action in cell 1 underscores how much suffering surgery is able to alleviate. Action in cell 4 points to the limits of surgery. It indicates how much is beyond the surgeon's skill and knowledge. Routine success and routine failure both have an air of inevitability which renders accounting unnecessary and which makes the extraordinary success or failure all the more conspicuous.

Confusing Situations

In terms of the sheer volume of cases, most action falls in cells 1 and 4. Cases in cells 2 and 3, unexpected success or failure, is much more rare. Because of their scarcity, these are professional events of some importance and at Pacific—as at most teaching hospitals—special ceremonies for the entire congregation of surgeons have evolved for witnessing them, resolving the confusion they create, and incorporating them into the group's history and the individual's biography. The fact that the marking of unexpected success or failure is a group ceremony of special importance is indexed by two facts. First, the two conferences in which they are discussed—Grand Rounds and the Mortality and Morbidity Conference—are the only occasions when all ranks and subgroupings of the Department of Surgery gather. And, second, they are the only occasions when work groups will put off tasks at hand—save operating, drop whatever they are doing, and attend a conference. As others have noted (Miller 1970), the houseofficer is faced with the dilemma of having to attend numerous confernces and provide patient care. The demands of both on his time cannot be satisfied and the individual adopts a short-run perspective which allows him to get by: he provides patient care and skips conferences. I also found this pattern—except for Grand Rounds and the Mortality and Morbidity Conference where the individual's normal accommodation is reversed. In surgery, all conferences wait until work is done, save these two. This is true for all ranks of the hierarchy. Attendings, as well as their underlings, feel compelled to attend and be on time. This punctual assembly of those accustomed to letting others cool their heels is quite remarkable. Schwartz (1974) has discussed waiting as an index of power of persons. Here punctuality testifies to the power of events.

What interests us about these meetings is the role attendings play in them. Attendings use these meetings to demonstrate their clinical wisdom which, as we noted, underlies their authority. The arbitrary elements of quick decisions justified only by rank and contradicted at times by scientific evidence are mitigated. By reserving for himself the right to resolve confusion, the attending legitimates his authority in these forums. The fact that unexpected success allows this is hardly surprising. However, that they are able to transform the negative experience of an unexpected failure into a positive one that serves as evidence of their wisdom is surprising and in need of some explanation. For the moment, suffice it to say that this satisfies the demands of the "heroic" element of the surgical role. The hero takes credit for his success but he is also able to accept the responsibility for his failures, to admit them openly, and to seek to remedy them. Through his trials, the hero learns the value of humility. As we have seen at the subordinate level, those who cannot behave with proper humility are seen as normatively wanting. This is also true at the attending level. In the following discussion of Grand Rounds and the Mortality and Morbidity Conference, we shall see how attending performance legitimates the application of everyday controls and how attendings use both meetings to demonstrate that they are worthy of the mantle of leadership since they accept its burdens along with its rights and privileges.

Cell 2: Unexpected Success—Grand Rounds

Grand Rounds celebrate the extraordinary successes of surgeons in cases where expectations are negative and outcomes are positive. In cell 2 of our chart we have ground-breaking success, such stuff as medical journal articles are made of. As we stated earlier, surgeons do not ordinarily operate with negative expectations. However, there are certain circumstances in which the presumption of success is suspended. Most commonly, two conditions make waiving the presumption of success warrantable. First, it is acceptable to waive the presumption of success when surgery is the only alternative left for a patient and it offers some hope, however slim, of salvaging the patient. Such situations inform the notion of the surgeon as hero.[5] Less glorious are cases where the patient's condition intersects with the surgeon's research in-

terests. At such times the surgeon rules out alternatives quicker
than usual and operates. Colleagues appreciate the courage,
judgment, and skill necessary to succeed in these situations.
Grand Rounds allow them to express this appreciation. Grand
Rounds also allow each attending the chance to demonstrate that
good reasons exist for the tyranny of his clinical judgment.

At a group level, Grand Rounds allow the entire collegium to
review the most recent successes of their colleagues and beyond
that the generalizable principles that are emerging for the surgical management of disease. As a weekly ritual, Grand Rounds
reconfirm for everyone that Pacific deserves its national reputation for excellence. At an individual level, Grand Rounds provide
attendings an arena to display their virtuosity. When questioned
about why they chose careers in academic medicine, attendings
invariably mention the importance of peer recognition:

> When I started medical school, I had the desire to be a
> surgeon. Surgeons were the most impressive guys, they got a
> lot of attention, they always seemed to be doing things. And
> I had a desire for all this; but the decision comes later when
> you graduate from medical school and you have all the train-
> ing before you. The training comes in two phases. In
> England, they are kept quite distinct, but here they are often
> intermingled. In the first phase, you must simply learn
> surgery: you have to learn techniques, pick up the basics. In
> the second phase, you have to learn judgment; you have to
> learn when to operate, when not to, and what operations to
> perform. And then when you finish, you have to decide if
> you're happy with this status or not. Now the "true" doctors
> who serve a community and are content to perform the
> common operations for the common conditions stop here.
> But there are those of us dissatisfied with this status who go
> into academic medicine. We want to do things that others
> can't. We want all the difficult cases referred to us. We want
> to train others to be good surgeons. We want to be recog-
> nized by our colleagues as an expert on some problem
> (Attending).

> Well, there are two aspects to that. One is, it's a real ego trip.
> You're surrounded by a small nucleus of people; and you're
> always patting each other on the back, telling each other how

great you are. Sometimes it's nothing more than a group of men playing children's games . . . the support of the peer group makes up for the financial sacrifices. So it's really a supportive atmosphere. It's gratifying to be at the top of the profession and have people tell you how good you are all the time. Second, although there are a lot of advantages to being in private practice—you can make more money, you can come home earlier, you have more free time—it can be very boring. You don't get the most interesting cases and you're surrounded by a lot of crap. Doctors who let patients die because they think that cancer is always incurable. You can really go out of your mind watching people practice bad medicine because they don't know any better. But here you can practice medicine in the highest quality circumstances. It's an ego trip. You pay heavily for it in terms of salary, administrative nonsense, long hours, family life, and personal life and leisure. A lot of it is really childish stuff but a lot of it feels really good. It's an ego trip to handle the toughest cases, to challenge yourself, and be among the best (Attending).

Grand Rounds provide an itinerary for the attending's ego trip; this conference assures that the peer recognition that attendings desire is provided in a fairly regular fashion. This recognition of skill comes in a much more direct and personal way than research publications provide. Of course, there are many other ways that colleagues pay homage to each other's skill. Informal consultation is one. More dramatic is when an attending acts as his colleague's first assistant. Here, he willingly subordinates himself to his equal, merely for the opportunity to watch the other work. Given the crowded nature of the attending's workday, such tributes are rare. When they occur, they highlight an aesthetic appreciation of flawless technique. Regularly scheduled, Grand Rounds are a device to distribute the amount of formal colleague support, approval, and recognition equitably. The rotation of the one to three cases presented weekly at Grand Rounds among services helps guarantee that the distribution of peer support is at least formally equal, despite whatever inequities evolve in the methods that colleagues informally grant approval.[6] Grand Rounds then serve to legitimate attending authority by demonstrating the high regard that attendings have for one another. For attendings, this regard is one of the primary rewards of the work environment.

More important, Grand Rounds allow attendings to model for their subordinates the proper way to accept their place in the medical elite. At the same time, this modeling is done in such a fashion to dramatize for subordinates the distance they must travel during training before they can claim to be equals. The standards of decorum that govern case presentation, the complete presentation of the clinical history, the review of the relevant literature, the elegant technique amply illustrated by slides of the operation, and their own restricted roles in the proceedings—all impress on subordinates the seriousness of the tasks before them, the accomplishments of their superordinates, and their own insignificance in bringing about these miraculous results. Grand Rounds model the virtuous performance of virtuous performance. The recurrent, almost invariant, mode of case presentation makes this modeling specific. First, subordinates present the clinical history of the patient. A good performance by a subordinate is one that as clearly and concisely as possible recounts an involved, complex clinical history. The subordinate gives a simple report, something which is not always a simple task. The subordinate is then for all practical purposes finished. He sits down and the superordinate takes over. First, the superordinate clarifies any ambiguity that arose during the subordinate's account. He then interprets the case history just presented. This interpretation routinely comprises a review of the clinical literature, a review which indicates that the attending's method for handling the case can improve the current mortality and morbidity rates. He adumbrates general principles which indicate that his results are replicable for all who would correctly apply his techniques.

But for one digression from professional and technical demeanor such an order of events would be entirely unremarkable. During the change of actors from subordinate to superordinate and the change of action from narration to interpretation the patient is often brought in and displayed for the group. Now, in some cases such as orthopedic ones, where the lame are literally made to walk, such presentations make sense; in most instances, however, the purpose is less clear as the group witnesses nothing more than a closed scar. The patient is asked a few questions about how he used to feel and how he feels now. Then he is led out. Once the patient is removed to the wings, the attending begins his exposition of the case. He renders a technical and learned account of the success. Case presentation lasts from thirty to forty-five minutes. The patient is present for generally less than three minutes.

These interruptions in what is for the most part very highly technical talk are striking for their brevity and their superficiality. Housestaff and attendings make jokes about the practice and complain that it serves no discernible purpose and that they learn nothing from it. Yet, if this is the case, why is this practice so regularly adhered to and why in those cases in which it is forgone is the attending presenting the case likely to include in his slide presentation a smiling snapshot or two of his cured patient?[7] First and most concretely, the patient is a living testimonial to the validity of the claims being made. Second, the interview with the patient shows the attending surgeon at his humanistic best. It allows him to demonstrate that alongside the technical expert about to teach a lesson, there is a humane healer who deals with the patient as a person. Third, the presence of the patient is gratifying for the attending. He is displaying one of the achievements he is most proud of, and he is in turn praised by his colleagues for this. Fourth, the introduction of the patient in the middle of the discussion reinforces group commitments by showing a case when the limits of the possible were extended. The whole group can share the sense of worthiness such patients inspire. The proud display of patients is a striking feature of Grand Rounds; however, display is limited to this conference. When patients who fall into cell 2 return to the clinic for follow-up visits, attendings round up as many subordinates and colleagues as possible for "ad hoc" displays:

I was in the clinic with Josh and Brian. They were writing charts in the work area when Arthur came in and told us all to go to examining room "D." There, Josh, Brian, and I were introduced to a patient. Arthur recited a brief history and invited an examination of his patient. Josh and Brian quickly examined the patient, nodded appreciatively, and then went about their tasks. Arthur thanked the patient and we left the room together. In the work area he turned to me and said: "That's why we're so demanding around here. By all rights that man should be dead. But there he is. That's the edge you get when you really bust your hump." He whistled to himself as he wrote a progress note in the patient's chart (Baker Service).

Finally, the last remark of Arthur's alerts us to what may be the most important feature of patient presentation. The display of past successes is an irrefutable argument to subordinates for the attending's hegemony. It is as if by this practice the attending tells his subordinate: "We can talk as equals when you have results like this to show off. Until then, respect the experience that achieves such results." Such displays of patients dramatize the distance between attendings and housestaff who do not have a ready stock of miraculous cures to parade.

Grand Rounds legitimate an attending's authority by dramatizing his most spectacular successes. Skill at presenting such cases is known as "roundsmanship"; it is a much appreciated skill. Those who have it are able to make the most of their extraordinary successes; and it is such ability that builds surgical reputations. Surgeons demonstrate this ability by elegantly explaining the extraordinary. Such performances dramatize the distance between them and their subordinates who, for whatever private praise they are given, are only allowed a very minor role in the proceedings.

Cell 3: Unexpected Failure—The Mortality and Morbidity Conference

It is not surprising that attendings use their extraordinary successes to legitimate the rigid hierarchical authority system of a surgical service. It is, however, noteworthy that they are able to use unexpected failure to serve the same end. In this section we explore the transformation of negative evidence into a positive display of an attending's skill. This transformation occurs in the Mortality and Morbidity Conference, in which cases that fall into cell 3—where expectations are positive and outcomes are negative—are discussed. The Mortality and Morbidity Conference is a form of retrospective peer review. The fact that attendings are able to use this forum to further consolidate their claims to authority is all the more remarkable when we consider that in this forum the attending's failures are presented for all to see and that this is the only occasion in surgical training that exists for public and open criticism of attending surgeons.

In the Mortality and Morbidity Conference the private understandings of failure achieved at the everyday level (chapters 2 and 3) are transformed into public knowledge. This transformation consists by and large of purging from the accounts the categories of normative and quasi-normative error and with them the implications of careless, lazy, negligent, or insubordinate performance they carry. At the Mortality and Morbidity Conference failure is accounted for professionally, that is, the reasons presented for it—with one notable exception—are formal and technical. In a sense this fact alone increases the power of the attending and further obligates his housestaff since the attending allows the knowledge of such substandard performance to remain a form of private, albeit guilty, knowledge.[8] Four factors account for the omission of normative and quasi-normative errors from discussion. First, such errors are an implicit indictment of an attending's control of his staff so it would ill serve him to publicize them. Second, attendings believe that if a subordinate makes a normative or quasi-normative breach on one service, he is likely to make them on others. There is no need to publicly humiliate subordinates; events will do so soon enough. Third, these errors are seen as indicative that unfit subordinates have character or personality disorders. There is little profit from exposing them since there is little hope of correcting them. Fourth, one purpose of the Mortality and Morbidity Conference is to illustrate that failure and error are an inevitable part of surgery and the best that one can hope for is to learn from these unfortunate hap-

penings so as not to be condemned to endlessly repeating them.
To introduce the scolding that accompanies normative and quasi-
normative errors into the Mortality and Morbidity Conference
would only encourage attempts to conceal complications. The
metapurpose of the conference would be destroyed if failure were
not treated as matter of factly as possible.

Like Grand Rounds, the Mortality and Morbidity Conference
has a remarkably consistent structure. However, the proceedings
have one more degree of freedom than do Ground Rounds, and it
is a very significant one. At the beginning of the meeting an
agenda is circulated.[9] The agenda lists the order of case presentation. The agenda provides the following information for each
case: the patient's age and sex, the service responsible for him,
the preoperative diagnosis, the procedures performed, and the
reason for presentation at the conference (either death or a specific complication). Also on the agenda is a record of the number
of major and minor operations performed by each service in the
preceding week. The agenda is a box score, and case presentation
is the play-by-play commentary. Case presentation is similar to the
format of Grand Rounds. The subordinate begins and gives a
case history. However, his job does not end here. He is on stage to
answer questions about the propriety of his behavior until either
his superordinate steps forward to give an interpretation of the
clinical history and an explanation of nodal choices, or until
another superordinate directs a question to his colleague. This
option of the attending to step forward or not is the degree of
freedom that the Mortality and Morbidity Conference possesses
that Grand Rounds do not. It is the exercise and use of this option
that allows attendings to transform a conference ostensibly about
their failure into a forum to celebrate their authority. We shall
now see how this is so.

The cases that are presented at the Mortality and Morbidity
Conference can be described in four basic ways. These are the
"normal troubles" of surgery. Each of these has its own accounting strategy. Two are relatively straightforward and do not
involve the attending playing a role in the proceedings unless
forced to. Two are relatively more complex and involve the at-

tending taking an active role in the accounting. In the first two cases it would be beneath the attending's dignity to explain failure where the causes are painfully obvious. In the latter two cases it would be beyond the houseofficer's skill to explain the failure, interpret the attending's strategy, and determine why events took the untoward turn they did.

The first and most simple case is when there is a routine complication easily managed after surgery. The complication is resolved without incident and, aside from the complication, the patient's recovery is uneventful. An example of such a case is a wound infection. For such cases accounting is as a rule solely the subordinate's responsibility.[10] Subordinates in this case align expectation and outcome by the claim that when all factors are taken into account—factors that were by their very nature unknowable before surgery—the outcome is really a success. The case belongs in cell 1 of our fourfold table. The argument that the complication notwithstanding the surgery was in fact a success hinges on the following claims: that although the rate of complication is known for a population at large, any individual occurrence cannot be predicted; that in this case sound prophylactic techniques have been applied but to no avail; and that once the complication presented itself, it was routinely and successfully treated. Such cases do not greatly arrest the attention of the conference's participants. So long as the subordinate clearly presents the case and competently answers a few questions, the case is quickly dispatched. Competently answering questions here means demonstrating that one knows what went wrong and why and that one has learned a lesson from this experience. The superordinate need not step forward since the patient's recovery as well as the thoughtful performance of his subordinate indicates that he is well aware of the situation and has it under control. The complications that are easily and quickly resolved are the ones that concern surgeons least, both in formal peer review and in everyday social control. In either circumstance, they are not seen as threats to competence but rather as routine and calculable parts of the environment.

The second straightforward case is the terminally ill patient and the questions his treatment provokes. When such patients are operated on, it is usually to palliate the more gruesome aspects of disease or to make a heroic attempt to rescue a trauma victim. The tactic of interpretation here is to have the expectation of success waived. The subordinate claims that the only reason that the service operated was because the situation provided no alternative, save the speedy signing of a death certificate. He claims that had the surgery been successful a miracle of modern medicine would have occurred. The case would have fallen into cell 2 of our table and have been appropriate for discussion at Grand Rounds. But since nothing of the sort happened, the patient was really without hope, and the case belongs to cell 4.

Straightforward as this accounting strategy is, it is not as readily acceptable to superordinates as the first tactic of interpretation outlined above. This is understandable if for no other reason than that death rather than recovery is the outcome in need of explanation. There are certain situations in which this accounting strategy is easily accepted by the audience. For example, there is the case of the trauma victim who receives multiple injuries and whose life is mechanically supported until the family decides if they will allow the cadaver to donate organs.[11] Another example is a patient operated on previously for the palliation of cancer's more gruesome sequelae who is successfully discharged and returns to the hospital some months later for terminal care because the family can no longer provide supportive care at home. Now, for such patients, ethical and philosophical questions may be raised: Did intervention add to or subtract from the patient's suffering? What is the relationship between the technical expertise we may demonstrate as surgeons and our humane responsibilities as healers? Though such questions are raised, they routinely serve to end discussion rather than begin it. In fact, those who raise questions about whether an operation was necessary or not often note that these questions are philosophical and inappropriate since the action has already occurred. Surgeons have a studied dislike for discourse on philosophical questions. They define such questions as endlessly debatable and, with their action ethic, surgeons have an almost trained incapacity to debate questions without answers. This is all the more so in cases where the patient's death is a certainty. Surgeons view debate here as unprofitable because "we know that exit is assured and all we would really be talking about is the mode" (Mortality and Morbidity Conference). Philosophic and ethical questions in this context signal members of the conference that, from the viewpoint of surgery as a scientific and value-free activity, they have nothing more to discuss. Moreover, attendings resist public discussions about the necessity of surgery and for good reasons. They fear publicly accepting any general principles for the limitation of effort. The internalization of such principles by the lazy, the unprincipled, or the inexperienced would, they feel, dilute the quality of care and provide an overly broad rationale for less than committed care. Noteworthy here is the contrast between the public silence of attendings at the conference and their private speech backstage on rounds about the limits of care and the treatment of the dying.

There are two situations in which the questions usually raised to end discussion begin it. The first of these is very rare. Attendings explain those cases which by all rights should have been the miraculous cures of cell 2, but which they chose instead to treat as the hopeless cases of cell 4. So extraordinary is such an event that it is set off from normal proceedings by the fact that the superordinate handles the presentation himself. He gives both the narration and exposition. He takes total responsibility. The subordinate plays no role in the proceedings at all.

> Dr. Porter, a pediatric surgeon, stepped forward to present the third case himself, mumbling as he walked to the front of the room, "I think I'd better take care of this myself." He began: "This third case is very different from the first two presented. Where the first two cases involve questions of patient selection and the taking of risk to prolong life, cases where everything must go right if the surgical intervention is to succeed, this third case involves the taking of risk not to prolong life. This is a decision that only an attending physician

can make and for which he alone is responsible. This infant
was born with 'prune belly' [wrinkling of skin on the belly
from absence of abdominal muscles], complete atresia of
the urethra [closing of outflow from urinary bladder], various
deformities of the legs and feet which may have been the
result of the fetus's position and may have been corrected
with time, an omphalocele [a large hernia at the umbilicus],
and a heart murmur. The obstetrician and the pediatrician
at the hospital where the infant was born put the baby aside
to die; but, as luck would have it, it did not. They then called
me up to arrange a transfer. They both expressed the hope
that the baby would die, but in my hands. Here is where the
situation gets complicated. The mother is a thirty-year-old
woman. She married at twenty-six and put off conception a
number of years while she was under psychiatric care. Then
she had some trouble conceiving and finally she had this
baby. She had never seen the child. The father, acting with
the obstetrician and the pediatrician, had arranged the
transfer and supported the decision not to make heroic efforts
to save the child's life. I thought we had to be straightforward
enough in this case to inform the mother of the baby's
problems and its chances because of the psychological
aspects of the mother-child, mother-father, doctor-patient
relationship, as well as our various legal responsibilities. So
I did the minimum necessary to give the baby a chance until
the mother could see it. I repaired the omphalocele. The
mother did come up and see the baby. She was obviously
under heavy sedation and quite difficult to deal with. She
waxed and waned in her support of the child. She couldn't
decide if the baby should survive. It was then that I decided
that the baby should not be considered for cardiac arrest
treatment, and that no urgent or emergency measures should
be taken to save the baby's life. These children need total
support if they are to have any chance at all. This baby would
never be normal and without the total support of both
parents there was no hope for a satisfactory adjustment. I
have seen many marriages totally disrupted by the extensive
hospitalization that such cases require after a number of
years. This is why I decided to let the infant die. This is, as
I said before, a decision that only an attending can make. It

is needless to say a very difficult decision. Yet in this case it
is one that I'm totally comfortable with" (Mortality and
Morbidity Conference).

After this presentation, no questions were asked. The attending's
right to make this decision and his grounds for doing so remained
unexplored. Rare as these cases are, they do establish what
considerations are used to establish the boundaries of effort.
Interesting here is the surgeon's definition of his client as the
entire family network; his interpretation of the Hippocratic
injunction, "First, do no harm"; and his weighing the quality of
life against the mere fact of life itself. The very extraordinariness
of this set of circumstances and the attending's public account of
his decision making show how firmly embedded the principle is
that the surgeon must do everything possible to prolong life.

This brings us to the second set of circumstances in which the
attempt to assign patients to cell 4 as a hopeless case raises rather
than ends questions for the audience. Here, the audience questions the subordinate's interpretation that the patient was in fact
a hopeless case. They challenge the subordinate's interpretation of the case as inevitable death. Such challenges are likely to
bring attendings in conflict with one another since it was the
attending in charge who more likely than not made most of the
management decisions with regard to the case and who has
discussed the cause of death and the case's presentation with the
subordinate onstage and on-the-spot at the moment:

> Andrew, a resident, had just explained that the death of an
> elderly lady following a gallbladder removal was caused by
> her old age and general physical weakness. He was imme-
> diately challenged by an attending. "That's not what I
> would call thinking real hard. I mean, you didn't exactly
> scratch your head until it bled on this one, did you, Andrew?
> You can't stand there and tell us this lady died from old age.
> If she was going to die from old age, why operate on her to
> begin with?" Dr. White, the attending on the case, rose to his
> resident's defense: "You're not exactly being fair. You know
> well enough that things like this can happen any time. It
> was just one of those unpredictable catastrophes." The other

attending answered: "That's bullshit. It doesn't sound like the
treatment of this lady was very well thought out." White
replied, "C'mon now, you have your share of cases like this.
She was a very strange old woman" (Mortality and Morbidity
Conference).

The attending's defense of his subordinate is a defense of
himself and his control over events. Beyond that, the attending
rescues the houseofficer from an uncomfortable situation. In so
doing he repays the subordinate for the indignities he subjects
him to in everyday situations. Such defenses are evidence of the
attending's authority and how it is used to shield as well as attack
subordinate performance.

You have to remember when something bad happens it's
usually at my instigation. Now, my orders may not have been
properly carried out. I may have ripped into the resident
before M&M. But I'm the responsible agent and I have to
back up my own people. You can't allow yourself to fall into
the syndrome of everything-that-goes wrong-is-the-resident's-
fault (Attending).

While disagreements may become as heated as the one above,
this rarely happens. The attending's support of his subordinate
and his assurance that everything possible was done is usually sufficient to quiet debate. So, despite the perturbations described
above, the strategy of having some failures redefined as cases that
fall into cell 4 is accomplished easily enough. This may be a
self-protective mechanism operating among attendings, an operative norm of reciprocity: if nobody pushes too hard, nobody will
be pushed too hard. Further, pushing too hard challenges the
deeply ingrained norm of individual responsibility for the patient
and is an affront to the decorousness of relationships among
colleagues.

The majority of the cases discussed at the Mortality and
Morbidity Conference are dispatched by the two tactics of interpretation discussed above. However, accounting for some failure
is relatively more complex. In these cases, the attending plays a
very important role in the proceedings and this role is an addi-

tional method for legitimating his authority. There are two types of problems that require this more complex method of social accounting.

In the first of these, surgeons must choose from among a number of procedures, none of which particularly recommend themselves. The probability of success for procedure A is the same as for procedure B or C and is in any case uniformly low. The surgeon must account for the procedure chosen when there are no clinically established protocols for it or any other procedure. These are the procedures that attendings at Pacific perform in order to maintain their standings as members of the national elite. Such cases are very important to attendings, they are evidence of their special place in medicine. Failure here disturbs the assumption that the attending's pride of place is deserved. This pride of place is, by the way, not a tacit background assumption but is right at the foreground of social consciousness, a constantly reiterated and well-articulated part of the work environment:

> The nurses on Baker Service were having problems with a patient. He was, in their opinion, irascible and they said they were tired of his addressing them in abusive tones. They complained to Dr. Grant, claiming it was not so much the patient's requests as the way he made them that bothered them. Dr. Grant answered: "Look—we will not put with this. We have all been under a lot of strain lately. You girls have been working particularly hard and we do not have to put up with an abusive patient. The way I look at it, we are doing Mr. Jameson a favor by operating on him—no other hospital around here would. He is an extremely poor operative risk. We do not promise our patients first-class hotel accommodations when they come here, nor do we promise them excellent cuisine. We only promise to get them better when no one else will treat them. It is we who are doing them a favor and not they us. This is really the same thing we went through with Michael Chometz. I'll talk with Mr. Jameson. And if he doesn't like what I say, then—fine! That is one less headache for us all" (Baker Service).

> Arthur had just operated on the wife of a close friend—her prognosis was poor, and he was complaining to me (he had

steered me to a corner where we were alone). "In academic
medicine you're motivated by the desire to be the best. That
means that you do a lot of cases that no one else would touch,
and that a lot of friends send their families to you. And while
I really hate the work, I'd hate it more if they thought someone else was better and they went to him. It's tough treating
these problems. Son of a bitch, it's the toughest part of
practice" (Baker Service).

Earlier, we noted that in such cases attendings need not prospectively justify their course of action to subordinates or colleagues. We noted that when their plans go awry there is no
everyday questioning such as they subject their housestaff to.
Such failures we coded as judgmental errors which we saw as a
privilege of rank. In the Mortality and Morbidity Conference
attendings pay for this privilege. They are obliged to explain how
eminences such as they made errors in judgment.[12] After the
subordinate's narration of the clinical history the attending steps
forward to field questions about the case. His taking over for the
subordinate indicates to his colleagues that the decisions in the
case were made by him and him alone, and that he alone will
answer for them. Difficult cases usually provoke a number of
questions from the audience, questions that are highly technical
in nature. For these cases, where a high degree of clinical uncertainty exists, the discussion reflects the academic and scientific
component of surgery. The conference becomes a seminar in
abstract problem solving. The longer the discussion continues,
the more complex it grows, the less subordinates participate, the
more discussion takes place among professional equals alone—
the attending surgeons. I shall hold off analyzing the attending's
account of the judgmental error until I have described the second
type of complex accounting situation since attending behavior is
similar in both of these situations.
   The other complex failure an attending must explain is the
failure of a statistically preferred treatment, especially when the
consequences of that failure are grave. Here the surgeon must face
the personal consequences of the statistical concept of variance.
In the first complex accounting situation, the working consensus
of the group momentarily disintegrates. Individual opinions

predominate. There is no consensus as to what proper treatment is. In the second situation—the failure of a preferred treatment—the working consensus of the group is highlighted. Instead of procedure-oriented concerns and scientific detachment, we find patient-centered and emotionally colored statements. The patient's age and social status are often invoked. Attributions about the patient often reflect the surgeon's feelings. They speak of "this poor, unfortunate teenage boy," or "this courageous mother of five," or "this unpleasant, unattractive alcoholic." During these accounts there is often a macabre and irreverent humor in which the whole group shares compared to the sombre discussion when treatment alternatives are unclear:

> Roger, a chief resident, was accounting for his decision to remove the hemorrhoids of a patient in the end stages of cancer. The patient had not been able to withstand this normally routine procedure and had bled to death. The wisdom of operating on a patient in such a compromised position was questioned. Roger replied: "He was in great pain from the hemorrhoids—he really was. Everyday on rounds he would beg us to do something for it. We agreed, but only reluctantly. But I can tell you one thing: When he died, he sure as hell died without pain from hemorrhoids." It was some time before order was restored (Mortality and Morbidity Conference).

Finally, when preferred treatments fail, the audience often offers supportive remarks to the surgeon involved, such as "We all have a few cases like this," or "It's a mystery to me." In extreme cases the moderator of the conference will place an arm on the shoulder of the speaker before he returns to his seat. In these cases, attendings also accept and publicly acknowledge their responsibility by taking control of the proceedings from their subordinates. How they use this control to dramatize the distance between themselves and their subordinates and to legitimate their authority is the topic we now turn to.

In both complex accounting situations, the major ritual that substitutes for the public sanctioning of attendings occurs. Attending surgeons publicly abase themselves before an audience

of their colleagues and subordinates. They publicly claim that
they made mistakes in the handling of the case. They put on the
hair shirt, as the argot of surgery has it. When an attending puts
on the hair shirt, he points out to the group what lessons he
learned from treating the patient; he explains why he might better
have followed some other course of action; and he urges all to
consider the case before acting on similar cases in the future. The
hair shirts the attending dons in each of these two complex accounting situations are slightly different from one another. In the
first type of case, the attending points out what clinical evidence
he in retrospect seems to have valued too little, that is, why he
made his miscalculation and how he will correct it in the future.

In the discussion of the death of a sixty-eight-year-old woman
on the cardiac service, the attending in charge of the case
said the patient's death presented two questions to him:
(1) should the woman have been operated on in the first place,
and (2) should she have been taken off antibiotics. He then
claimed that the patient's death indicated that he was wrong
for deciding to operate in the first place. He then lectured
the group on the parameters one must evaluate in choosing
to operate or not (emphasizing as he did the parameter whose
importance he paid too little attention to). This finished,
he gave a similar lecture on the use of antibiotics (Mortality
and Morbidity Conference).

Two infant deaths were presented by the pediatric surgery
service. Both cardiac patients with similar problems were
presented at the same time. After the recital of the two
clinical histories, the attending in charge took over. He discussed the technical problems involved in handling the case
and what research needed to be done before one could hope
to successfully treat these patients. Then he claimed that
"as it stands now anybody that comes to me with this problem
already has their ticket punched"—a reference to the inevitability of death. He then gave a very short speech about how
both patients were very young infants and how these young
infants accounted for almost all the mortality among pediatric
cardiac patients. He claimed that such patients represented
the greatest challenge in the field and that he hoped the next

generation of surgeons would be able to solve these problems and wonder how come his generation lost all these cases. His presentation lasted six minutes and no questions were asked (Mortality and Morbidity Conference).

With this hair shirt, the attending demonstrates for his subordinates the behavior that he expects when they make lesser technical and judgmental errors. He shows how he has reconsidered his behavior as the emerging events brought them into question and he shows what lessons such reconsiderations have brought home to him.

The second type of hair shirt demonstrates a different type of expected behavior from subordinates, that is, total integrity and complete disclosure of shortcomings rather than any attempt at cover-up. In the second type of case, when an attending puts on the hair shirt he grounds the failure in his improper supervision of his subordinates. Attendings believe that these are deaths and complications that should just not occur and when such misadventures do occur, they blame themselves for their own lack of foresight. While privately they damn their subordinates for what they see as treacherous behavior for a physician, attendings publicly state that it was their negligence and not that of their housestaff that accounts for the failure:

> After the case of Mr. Will was presented, Arthur sprang from his chair and said that he had a few words to say in the matter. He said: "I think that this case represents all the things that are wrong with the hierarchy of a teaching hospital. Here we have one of society's unfortunates. Mr. Will came to us with no kith or kin. He was comatose when he arrived and we still really don't know who Mr. Will is or why he came to us. The first in the comedy of errors made on this man was made by the medical service. The decision by them not to dilate his abdomen was tantamount to gross neglect. I only mention the medical service because they are here and because I'm now going to turn to the errors we made in treating this man. First, I made a fundamental error this early in the training year in allowing the chief resident to operate solo in this emergency. We should have

learned from experience never to do this. In our defense we
discussed this case with the resident involved over the phone.
The third guilty party is the chief resident involved. By not
calling for help when he ran into trouble, the resident took
undue risk with the patient's life. Fortunately, the case looks
like it will have a happy ending because of some heroic efforts made to undo the damage. Now, Mr. Will is an old,
unattractive, abandoned, cirrhotic black man whom we
almost abandoned to surgical pathology. Our surgical responsibility rests evenly with our unattractive as well as our more
attractive patients. In this case, we have clearly committed
surgical immorality." When he finished, no one spoke
(Mortality and Morbidity Conference).

After the presentation of a case in which there had been a
complication from the insertion of a subclavian catheter, Dr.
Stone rose to speak: "This case is unfortunate and represents a want of supervision on my part. Clearly, this is a
simple error in technique that could have been avoided if
the resident had had proper instruction. The insertion of a
subclavian catheter can be a very tricky business. It requires
poise and confidence. It should be carefully supervised. Unfortunately, it is one of those procedures that we are least
likely to monitor. All too often, we instruct our residents to
insert subclavian catheters as we walk off the floor on our
way home for the night. We should not—as I did in this
case—do this. We should make sure our subordinates are
properly equipped to do this and we should be there to provide help until we are confident our housestaff can do these
things on their own. It is our responsibility to be available
and provide instruction. We cannot always count on our
housestaff to properly assess the trickiness of techniques"
(Mortality and Morbidity Conference).

In the first type of account, the attending takes total responsibility for all decisions and for the way that they were carried
out. He indicts his judgment in handling the case. In the second
case, he takes responsibility for decisions, even maintains they
were correct, but tries to separate himself from the way the
decisions were carried out. He does not totally excuse his sub-

ordinates but blames himself for allowing their performance to proceed unchecked. If the subordinate makes a mistake it is only because his superordinate allowed him to do so. On the face of it, this is quite an admission for an attending to make; it is tantamount to the confession of a normative error. The attending tells all assembled that his commitment to patient care was wanting and some patient was caused unnecessary suffering. The only redeeming feature of this confession is that it sets a standard for full and open disclosure and complete intellectual integrity that houseofficers are expected to match. In either case, when an attending puts on a hair shirt he admits error, points out the lessons in it, and urges all to consider these before hasty action in the future. Attendings wear a hair shirt because a death or complication, especially when unexpected, is a pretty damning piece of evidence that forces them to consider alternatives. However, that they so willingly admit error and humble themselves before a group of colleagues and subordinates seems strange. How are we to account for this practice which seems to run against the grain of human nature, which usually conceals, minimizes, and denies error?

Two factors seem most noteworthy. First, as attendings often state, one purpose of the Mortality and Morbidity Conference is to instill professional "superegos" in junior staff. When an attending puts on the hair shirt, he makes the working of his own professional superego transparent. He shows what considerations should inhibit a too hasty impulse to act. Second, these public confessionals serve to mitigate the rigid hierarchical authority system of a surgical service. When he dons the hair shirt, the superordinate humbles himself before an audience of many subordinates over whom he has complete career control and whom he chews out daily. The conference is the only occasion when an attending is open to criticism. That this is self-criticism rather than the more acrimonious and harder to bear ill judgment of others is important but beside the point. These public ritualized admissions of fallibility contrast sharply with the everyday behavior of attending surgeons and serve to mitigate it somewhat.

This interpretation of the hair-shirt ritual is given greater plausibility when we consider additional aspects of the practice. The humbling effects are ordinarily softened, either by other attendings who indicate that they would have handled the case in the same way or who cite similar examples from their own clinical history or by pathologists who indicate that the patient was ravaged by disease and beyond repair. More interestingly, "wearing the hair shirt" is a prerogative of status. Although junior staff are forced to wear the garment in the informal setting of rounds (in fact, having thought through a death or complication, admitting responsibility, and pointing out the clinical lesson learned is one of the ways they establish that they are competent and trustworthy), they are not allowed to wear the hair shirt in the public conference. In these cases, the breach between expectation and outcome is not satisfied until the attending offers his exposition of events. Even though a subordinate may know the facts of a matter, he cannot authoritatively resolve the confusion these facts create.

The attending's refusal to let subordinates wear the hair shirt in public is an attempt by senior surgeons to illustrate to junior surgeons what the acceptable limits of a professional superego are. Attendings want subordinates to be mindful of the consequences of their action; however, they do not want them to be overly scrupulous. They do not want excessive thought—an overestimation of risk—to inhibit clinically indicated action. By refusing to allow subordinates to blame themselves for certain failures, attendings show that professional second-guessing properly ends where professional authority ends. In so doing, they once again underscore the status differences among their ranks. There is a very subtle give-and-take going on in the Mortality and Morbidity Conference. On the one hand, attendings encourage subordinates to question the grounds for their action; yet on the other, attendings try to limit that questioning so that it does not impair the quick judgments necessary in surgery.

There is yet another reason why "wearing the hair shirt" is a privilege of rank; it would be unseemly in a junior surgeon. If a junior surgeon claims he is mistaken often enough, we must take him seriously. At this point in his career, when competence is always an issue, weekly self-incriminations would ill serve the junior surgeon. Also, the hair shirt might prove too attractive for the subordinate. He might wish to wear it too often and therefore not be self-critical enough to see how his performance can be improved, or he may never learn to discriminate between those failures which he can and cannot control. An unrestrained *mea culpa, mea culpa* ill fits the heroic ideal of grace under pressure into which surgeons are socialized. Now, this is not so for the attending surgeon who stands at the top of his profession. He has a luminous professional biography and history—his credentials are unshakeable. The cases in which he assumes responsibility are marginally worthless in assessing his competence. These pale in comparison to his great achievements. In fact, for the super-ordinate, putting on the hair shirt only emphasizes the surgeon's charity, humanity, and the scope of his wisdom. It allows him to round out his professional self by adding to it the secondary qualities associated with the healer in our culture: humility, gentleness, wisdom, and a certain wry acceptance of the universe that allows him to accept the limits of human activity. It allows him to express guilt without being consumed by it. Such expressions of guilt might consume the subordinate who does not yet have the same mastery. It is difficult to adopt a long-run perspective and be philosophical without the stock of experience that encourages such wisdom. By allowing actions that cause guilt to be openly confessed, putting on the hair shirt is a form of institutionalized self-protection for attendings. At the same time, it communicates to subordinates that no one is perfect; it models for them the proper expression of guilt and teaches them to accept that such accidents are an inevitable, unfortunate, and intractable fact of professional life:

> The conference is for the housestaff really. First, we go
> through the dialogue to point out verbally, schematically, and
> theatrically the issues involved. It is a teaching device first
> and foremost. Second, it shows by example honesty and lack
> of immunity from the problems of the profession. It teaches
> that these problems will be with them their whole professional
> life. Third it's good for our own characters to admit mistakes.

Deaths and complications are great levelers in surgery. It
teaches that you are not the archangel Gabriel, that you
bleed when cut (Attending).

Putting on the hair shirt is the major and most striking activity
of formalized retrospective peer review. By this practice surgeons
excuse their mistakes by admitting them. The major punishment
of the practice is the embarrassment of a public confessional and
the pain the outcome itself actually causes the surgeon's conscience. As a form of social control, this admission of error rests
on the self-surveillance and self-reports of the individuals involved. In this sense, it is part of a chivalrous code of behavior.
Moreover, when an individual can wear the hair shirt, he has
more or less passed beyond the few available social controls
surgery has. So this is a hair shirt on the outside only; for the
wearer it has the silken lining of unconditional professional support. Nevertheless, it is proper to ask how common it is for
attendings to avoid this public embarrassment and to conceal
their failure and what the consequences of this behavior are.

The actual extent of concealment is difficult, if not impossible,
to measure. On Able and Baker Services we never observed such
activity. Yet all subordinates are able to recall cases when services
they were on absented themselves from the conference at strategic
points. Both superordinates and subordinates take a dim view of
such behavior; and although all agree it occurs, they also agree its
actual extent is rare. When such behavior is even suggested it is
met with severe distaste:

Paul asked Mark if Carlos's wound infection was on this
week's Mortality and Morbidity agenda. Mark replied: "Of
course." A student asked: "Why did you do that? You
schedule the cases yourself. You know that there's no one
looking over your shoulder to check out what should be at
M&M." Mark answered sharply: "That would be no good. A
physician that doesn't own up to his own mistakes is no better
than the shit that's draining out of Carlos's wound. No, this
leak in the anastomosis is clearly a technical error. I still
don't know what caused it. It could have been caused by any
of a multitude of factors. But it is our error. No doubt about

it, and we're going to have to take our lumps for it" (Able Service).

Sure, a few complications are hidden by senior staff. I know of three right now. It's predictable behavior from the individuals involved. It's a case of insecurity leading to weakness and weakness leading to dishonesty. The individuals involved are destroyed by this. They lose all credibility and professional respect (Attending).

The refusal of superordinates to wear the hair shirt is a serious breach, comparable to the lack of total disclosure attendings demand from housestaff. Those attendings who do not wear the hair shirt often enough or who, worse yet, conceal their complications, undermine their own authority with colleagues and subordinates.[13] Wearing the hair shirt and scrupulously reporting all operative misadventures serves as evidence to subordinates that an attending applies to his own work the same standards he applies to theirs. It serves as evidence to colleagues that he respects the highest professional ideals and is ready to sacrifice face to protect them.[14] An attending that is publicly honest and open about his own shortcomings earns the right to be arbitrary, stubborn, and dogmatic on occasion because his own integrity and motives are beyond question. He has demonstrated that he is dedicated above all to the improvement of patient care.

five

Climbing the
Pyramid:
Professional
Control and
Moral Identity

So far our discussion of social control in a surgical training program is incomplete. We have analyzed how blameworthy failure is discovered and distinguished from blameless failure. We have seen what surveillance techniques attendings use to determine who guilty parties are and how guilty they are. We have analyzed the dramaturgic legitimation of the considerable authority that allows an attending to act as a houseofficer's defender and/or prosecutor at the same time that he is his judge. Yet so far this discussion neglects the enduring punishments superordinates impose on subordinates while emphasizing such obvious and immediate disciplinary tactics as verbal scorn, public ridicule, and icy and contemptuous avoidance. In this chapter I remedy this defect by extending our temporal perspective from the recurrent everyday level to the longer-run perspective of the fifteen-month period in which a cohort of subordinates is evaluated. As we move conceptually from the level of incident to the level of biography we shall see that attendings do more than get angry at erring houseofficers, they also exert a most powerful influence on an individual's career path. At the end of a subordinate cohort's first fifteen months of training, attendings decide which houseofficers will be allowed to complete their surgical training at Pacific, which will be forced to pursue careers at less elite institutions, and which will be advised to give up surgical careers altogether. Attending surgeons make these gate-keeping decisions at a faculty meeting of the Department of Surgery. This meeting—or meetings, if the decisions are particularly difficult to make—is the last time subordinates are judged formally as a group.[1] It is a nodal moment in a surgical career and it goes without saying that it warrants our careful consideration. In this chapter, we give a brief description of the context that surrounds the attending's decision making, show how attendings apply a "value-added" logic to evaluate houseofficers, and demonstrate that the promotion decision is a presumptive moral licensing that provisionally admits or blackballs a subordinate from the fraternity of academic surgeons.

The Context

The surgical training program at Pacific is a "pyramid" program. Each year more interns are accepted than there are places for senior residents. Part of this surplus is planned for. These are interns with a primary interest in one of the surgical specialties, such as orthopedics or urology, who must gain some experience in basic surgical techniques before they enter the subspecialties. The remainder of the interns are those who hope to advance to the top of the pyramid. In the year for which we made our observations, six people competed for four slots. The number of slots was, however, negotiable, and in fact only three positions were filled. The attendings at Pacific chose to operate with one empty slot rather than either accept one of their own subordinates whom they found wanting, or submit to the organizational humiliation of filling a position with an intern who had failed to climb the pyramid at some other elite institution. The fact that attendings were willing to fill only three positions despite funding for a fourth is very significant. It indicates how seriously they take their "gate-keeping" functions; attendings were not willing to compromise standards merely because the budget allowed it.

The decision to leave a position empty caused much debate. The attendings originally voted to fill four slots. Two factors were decisive: such staffing had been the tradition of the program, an expectation that subordinates had been laboring under for the last fifteen months and, more important, an increased case load was anticipated for the following year. There were many reasons for this expectation. First, there was a "maturing" of the faculty. There was a recent increase in the number of attendings at Pacific and these new attendings were building their practices quickly. Second, efforts were under way to make the referral of more difficult cases from community hospitals to Pacific more formal and more efficient. There was some resistance to these colonizing efforts by the community hospitals but it seemed clear to all attendings that much progress had been made. Legislation making programs for continuing medical education compulsory in such community hospitals served to strengthen the position of the attendings at Pacific and increase their optimism. However, after the attendings surveyed the second-year crop of subordinates and found it wanting and after they decided it was unwise to allow a member of the first-year group to skip a rank, the attendings reversed their original decision and filled only three positions. After reaching this decision, a number of attendings expressed some relief that the closing of the state-run facility to which they were committed to providing coverage offered a convenient "PR" reason for closing ranks unexpectedly. By this public or official reason, these attendings hoped to sidestep the unpleasantness that a direct confrontation with the real reason—a shortage of residents with acceptable skills—would have necessitated. Facing the real reason squarely was painful to attendings who may have had to revise cherished notions about their own and the department's preeminence in the field and painful to subordinates who may have had to revise notions about their own worth.

Since such a weighty matter was not easily resolved, analyzing the questions it raised tells us much about Pacific as an institution. The issues discussed by the attendings in resolving this staffing problem reveal many of their concerns as medical educators. The question of the very steepness of the pyramid itself was raised as a general concern. The attendings felt that too steep a pyramid would encourage an unhealthy competition which would undermine the teamwork necessary for a high level of care. All attendings recalled with horror past times when the pyramid had grown too steep and it was difficult to obtain cooperation among residents. On the other hand, the faculty feared that a too gently sloping pyramid discouraged one external incentive for high-quality performance. Proper staffing was a mechanism for encouraging and restraining competition. Next, there was the question of what number of residents was consistent with the program's primary goal of training high-quality academic surgeons. With overstaffing at the senior levels, the danger exists that each senior resident does not get his share of emergencies and challenging cases and so is unprepared for all the contingencies he must face when released from training. Moreover, if standards were compromised to admit staff to senior ranks of training, attendings complained that the effort necessary to make the less-qualified competent is taken from the effort necessary to make the more-qualified superior. Attendings were convinced that such a trade-off was inconsistent with the training program's present reputation and goals as well as its future pretensions. Also, attendings questioned what number of senior residents was proper to insure that each of them would have an intense enough relationship with their apprentices to assure that he would have an impact on a houseofficer's thinking and his career. Such a consideration is very important to attendings for they feel that those they train and brand with their personal stamp contribute to their own personal reputation as well as the organization's. Some attendings state that those they train are in the long run more important than their research or clinical contributions:

> I was talking to Dr. Grant. It was late in the afternoon and we were alone in the doctor's lounge. He said: "Are you going tonight to hear Dr. Daily of Eastern Hospital speak? You really should, you know. You can learn a lot from seeing him. He is a very distinguished surgeon—one of the most creative surgeons in America. You can learn a lot from seeing him. You know, he has never trained anyone of prominence. And in academic surgery that is what counts most—whom you have trained. Long after your research is forgotten and your papers are outdated, people will remember you by whom you have trained. And Daily has trained no one—at Eastern—where he gets the pick of the top talent. You know why? He can't work with residents. He has to compete with them. He has to dominate them. And he winds up crushing them. Go hear him talk. He can tell you a lot about surgery" (Baker Service).

The debate over how many positions to fill is, for attendings at Pacific, a much more complex problem than arriving at the proper solution to an equation balancing the demand for services and the supply of servers. It is also a debate about what members see as the character of their institution and its proper mission. At Pacific attendings regulated the supply of servers mindful of, but not contingent on, the demand for services. Such a stance was one they felt was consistent with the training program's primary goal, producing surgeons capable of making both academic and clinical contributions. It is easy enough to imagine how other hospitals of a different order than Pacific may see staffing more narrowly as a supply-demand problem. For example, community hospitals whose primary mission is to provide service might determine the number of residents more with an eye to anticipated case load and local market considerations than the attendings at Pacific, who can within limits regulate demand by refusing less interesting referrals and accepting only those minor cases necessary to fulfill the program's need to provide cases for the less experienced.

Despite the debate over how many positions to fill, when it got down to cases the decision to promote or not was made independent of the original understanding to fill four slots. So when it turned out that the attendings felt that they had only three qualified residents, they reversed their original decision to staff four positions. Had there been five qualified residents, then I feel that the attendings would have been reluctant to lose a good prospect. Before the discussion of individual cases, attendings reminded each other that the training program had a great deal of built-in flexibility and that should there be a surfeit of qualified residents in the group, they had a number of options. For example, a resident could be asked to step out of the queue and work on a laboratory project and then return to the program at a later date. Just as there was no need to accept the unqualified because of excessive demand, there was no reason to reject the qualified because of a temporary embarrassment of riches. On a whole, it seemed that the immediate needs of the organizational environment exerted less influence on the decision-making process than did longer-run commitments to professional excellence.

Given this commitment to professional excellence, how is it determined in any particular case whether an individual is

qualified or not? Attendings evaluate the performance of subordinates in written recommendations. These letters are entered
in a subordinate's personnel file and are the official record of
his performance. In the fifteen-month period before decision
making, a subordinate will rotate through between eight and
twelve services. Each of these services is run by two or three
attendings. So, for the time period involved, subordinates ac-
cumulate approximately twenty-four letters of recommendation.
These letters range in length from a simple letter grade to a few
words to a few paragraphs. They also vary considerably in
specificity. Only one resident evaluation of the over 100 we
perused mentioned a specific incident critical or supportive of
a resident's performance. More commonly, letters will speak in
generalities. They will state that a resident has "some difficulty
getting along with staff or other residents," or that "there is fairly
common friction between this resident and nurses," or that "he is
still occasionally bothered by personality conflicts with his co-
workers," and not mention what these difficulties are. Letters of
praise are likewise very vague, often stating nothing more about a
resident than that "he is outstanding in every respect," or that
"he should have a very promising career."

These evaluations of resident performance are interesting
documents in their own right. They indicate how very consequential typifications are made and supported by only the merest
shards of evidence. These evaluations illustrate the various
interpretive procedures by which performance and performers
are labeled. There is labeling by analogy, that is, statements of
the type that "at this stage in his training, X reminds me of Y"
(where Y is an old resident). There is labeling by hypothesis, that
is, statements of the type, "I expect a person like X to perform in
such and such a fashion if confronted by situation Y." There is
labeling by negative or positive hyperbole, that is, statements of
the type that "this resident is so bad or good that words cannot
describe his performance." There is labeling by elliptical allusion, that is, statements of the type that allude to a specific
problem that a subordinate has without ever providing an
example. All these techniques indicate that labeling does not

proceed through a careful sifting and documentation of cases, but through artfully employed rhetorical devices. One reason that careful documentation is unnecessary is the respect that attendings have for each other's clinical wisdom. The rhetorical devices of analogy, hypothesis, hyperbole, and allusion are a shorthand language that all colleagues understand, share, and employ to describe what are very complex judgments of performance. The nature of the evaluations is itself prima facie evidence of the importance of clinical judgment and the attendings' claims to it. Were this not so, efforts would be made to make the evaluations more standardized, rendering them more comparable and replicable, that is, scientific.

Be that as it may, these evaluations are, for our purposes, not very useful. They show us what kinds of facts about house-officers attendings find worthy of recording. They show us how everyday experience is generalized. But the documents in and of themselves tell us little about the decision-making process of promotion. To understand this, we have to look to the dynamics of the promotion meeting itself. We have to analyze the decision making and not the documents that are invoked as a background resource to justify a particular decision.

Value-Added Logic and Sorting

At the promotion meeting when attendings evaluate each resident's performance, they have three options before them: (1) they can decide that no amount of training will ever make a resident a competent surgeon and recommend that he try another speciality; (2) they can decide that, while a resident will in all likelihood become a competent surgeon, he lacks the wherewithal to serve in an elite atmosphere, and recommend that he try another training program; (3) or they can decide that a resident is competent and admit him to the ranks of senior residency. The attending problem is to sift through the available talent and sort it. Superordinates discipline subordinates in the long run by excluding them from their professional networks and they reward them by including them. The main mechanism of social control is sorting.[2]

Sorting as a process involves ordering what would otherwise be a chaotic congregation of elements by categories and then within categories, subcategories. As a process, sorting operates within a value-added logic (Smelser 1962), that is, the result of each sort narrows the range of possible outcomes for the next sort. In evaluating residents and thus setting their career options, attendings apply such a value-added logic. This logic is appropriate to their task at hand—putting each subordinate in his proper place.[3] As the work of Bittner (1967) on police discretion and Cicourel (1969) on juvenile justice show, sorting is a standard operating procedure for social control agents. Sorting is applied typification. Moreover, value-added sorting is a basic socially structured cognitive process which we all use to order, name, and thereby behave appropriately in social situations. Our task here is not to account for the basic process, but to show how attendings employ it to rank subordinates and exercise professional control.

The first sorting question is, Does an individual possess the technical capacity to be a surgeon? Two of the six individuals in the cohort I observed were judged as lacking the motor skills and the temperament necessary for surgery. Such determinations were arrived at quickly:

> "The next person on our list is Smith," said Dr. Gray, the department chairman. Dr. White comments: "He was a mistake. I think we should advise him to take a career in something other than surgery. I'm surprised he's on this list. I thought I had convinced him six or seven months ago to go into another specialty." Dr. Peters: "He's an absolute clunker. He has no promise." Dr. Pines: "He should be in another specialty." Dr. Ross: "There is absolutely no hope of training him to be a competent surgeon." Then Dr. Gray says, "Okay. Then we are all agreed. I'll talk to Smith and see if we can work something out for him. Perhaps in one of the other departments here" (Department Meeting).

The faculty were agreed that Smith lacked the requisite skills necessary to be a surgeon at any institution, but despite this, they were not willing to banish him from the ranks of the elite altogether. What happened in his case was on each service that he rotated through he made technical errors and failed to improve over time. This was evidence for all that he could never be a surgeon. However, on each service, Smith handled these errors in a proper fashion. He recognized them quickly, reported them, and made certain they were corrected. His repeated misadventures convinced his superordinates he lacked talent as a surgeon. Nevertheless, his normative propriety convinced his superordinates that, although Smith was in the wrong field, he might be in the right place. They were ready to counsel him and recommend him to colleagues in other departments at Pacific. The attendings viewed Smith as a simple tracking problem: he had the intelligence and integrity necessary to be a member of the medical elite and attendings concerned for his welfare wanted to see him placed properly. Their willingness to help Smith was encouraged by Smith's growing sense that he had made an error in choosing a surgical career, by his willingness to discuss this openly with attendings, and by his eagerness to work out more viable options.

The faculty agreed as quickly as they did in Smith's case that a second candidate, Jones, lacked the technical skills necessary for a surgical career. But in this second case, they had grave doubts about whether Jones had any place in the medical profession at all. Jones had combined technical maladroitness with an inability to admit mistakes and difficulties in communicating with patients and staff. This had led on occasion to small correctable errors growing into catastrophes.

> Dr. Gray opened discussion of Jones by reporting: "Jones has had a lot of problems over the last fifteen months. This morning, I talked with him and told him that an inability to communicate with peers and patients was not a quality we were looking for in our residents. I suggested to him that he meet with Dr. Cantor in psychiatry to discuss whatever personal problems he has before he makes any plans to continue his career in any capacity. He was quite adamant that he needed no help and that he wanted to be a surgeon."
> Dr. Grant said: "I did not know what to make of Dr. Jones

his first few days on our service, but I have reluctantly come to
the conclusion that this man is sick. I don't trust him around
my patients." An attending asked, "How do you mean sick—
physically or mentally?" Dr. Arthur answered, "Mentally. He's
off his rocker. Totally out to lunch. He needs help and he
needs it quick. The question is not whether we should keep
him, but whether he should finish out the year. In my mind, I
wonder if he's on drugs." Dr. Gray then said: "As I said before
when I gave him the option of seeing Dr. Cantor, he was totally
opposed to it." Dr. Grant added: "There is no doubt he needs
help. Yesterday in clinic he was really around the bend. He
couldn't focus on patients. You could not have a conversation
with him. He couldn't deal with anything." Dr. Peters commented that "it doesn't sound like much has changed over the
course of a year. Maybe he has a brain tumor." Dr. Ross said:
"If he has a problem, I don't think we could in good conscience
let him go without offering him help. I think we have a
responsibility to see that he gets proper care. But our responsibility to our patients comes first. If there is doubt about his
stability, we cannot continue to let him see patients." Dr. Gray
then summarized the comments about Jones by saying: "Then
we are agreed. Not only will Jones not be offered a position,
but he will not be allowed to return to duty until he is investigated by someone in neuropsychiatry" (Meeting).

The attendings felt some responsibility for Jones as a person
under their care. However, Jones' breaches were so consistent and
so consistently denied by Jones that immediate expulsion was
necessary. Unlike Smith, Jones was not a tracking problem. He
was a total problem that attendings wished to rid themselves of
entirely by shifting responsibility to the psychiatry department.

The contrast between the handling of Smith and Jones supports my argument about the differences between technical and
normative error and also suggests inherent limits to professional
control. A lack of requisite technical skill disqualifies one for a
surgical career but not for a career as a physician. If one has made
a mistake in choosing to be a surgeon, and if that mistake is
compounded by acceptance in a surgical training program, it can
be corrected. The cost of the mistake is the time the subordinate

spent in training and the effort superordinates wasted trying to teach him. However, as long as the subordinate complies with the norms of his role, the cost to patients is kept at a minimum. Moreover, while the subordinate's performance demonstrates to his superordinates that he will never be a surgeon, at the same time it convinces them that in the proper field he has a contribution to make. The problem is wedding aptitudes and inclinations to the proper clinical area. On the other hand, an absence of technical and normative skills indicates to super-ordinates that an individual is unfit to be a physician. Unfortunately, such knowledge comes too late. The subordinate has already graduated from medical school. He is a doctor. Super-ordinates as agents of professional control can block some career options. They can suggest that an individual get help. But they cannot block all career options. Nor can they force an individual to seek help. Their jurisdiction is limited. If they are willing to take enough trouble, they can perhaps block training in many institutions. But there are internships that go abegging every year; and, ironically, failing at Pacific may recommend an individual to a more lackluster organization. A sufficiently stubborn individual can get trained and eventually licensed to practice medicine, even if he has to give up his ambition to be a board-certified surgeon. Attendings know that there is nothing that they can do to stop this. They realize the market for medical school graduates is highly differentiated. In some sectors, it is a buyer's market; in others, it is a seller's. This split-market structure does much to frustrate attendings' efforts at control.

The four remaining candidates passed the first "sort," that is, it was agreed by all attendings that these residents possessed the technical skills necessary for careers as surgeons. The second sorting question concerns a person's "teachability," that is, his ability to learn from his mistakes and improve on his performance. Attendings ask, Will this person mature? They use three indicators for this: a resident's relations with patients and nurses, his general level of enthusiasm, and his relationship to and with attending authority. Of the four residents who passed the first sort, three passed the second. There was little disagreement about the three candidates that passed the second sort; consensus was quickly reached. On the other hand, much controversy surrounded the fourth candidate. He was debated over one hour at the first promotion meeting. The attendings were not able to come to any decision regarding his future, and scheduled a second meeting to continue discussion. Discussion at the second meeting lasted over two hours. At the end of this meeting, the attendings declined to offer the resident a position. Before discussing this long debate, it is helpful to look at the decision to retain the other three residents. This will provide us a useful contrast.

Consensus to keep the three qualified residents was quickly arrived at. No attending mentioned any problem that arose and recurred with any of the three residents. Discussion started with a statement of praise for the resident. This was echoed by an attending from a second service and then from a third. After the third attending spoke, others nodded their agreement. Gray, seeing that his colleagues were of one mind, then announced: "Okay, we're agreed. We'll keep him." In the first promotion meeting, which lasted three hours, only fifteen minutes, more or less, were spent discussing all three promoted residents. A typical exchange went as follows:

> Dr. Gray: "Okay, Thomas is next." Dr. Arthur: "Top-drawer. He's very quiet, but also very resourceful with patients, who like him a lot." Dr. Peters: "Yes, we were quite pleased with his work on our service. He works hard and he's very conscientious." Dr. Ross: "His growth has been very good. He reminds me of Stone at a similar stage in his career, and as his confidence grows he may—like Stone—become less quiet." Dr. Gray, summarizing: "This boy is a real sleeper. I get the impression from looking over his folder that our opinion of him has grown with each rotation. We're agreed to keep him" (Meeting).

Residents are accepted to Pacific with high expectations for their performance based on their stellar records as medical students. For the three residents promoted to the senior ranks, these positive expectations were satisfied. The performance of these residents serves as testimony to the wisdom of accepting them in the first place. Nothing much really needs to be said about them.

This is not so for the resident who on occasion displays great technical prowess combined with normative lapses. Attendings have difficulty in accounting for his failure to meet expectations, and difficulty in deciding what to do with him. Of this resident attendings are forced to ask, Can we make him change, and does his promise justify the high cost in terms of time and energy necessary to work this change? This is a difficult decision to arrive at for a number of reasons. Chief among these is the fact that attendings recognize that it is the very qualities which cause one to be vexed with and disappointed in subordinates that may allow one to be a creative and outstanding member of the medical elite. Brashness, aggressiveness, and even stubbornness are qualities that can make a subordinate insufferable and lead him to make normative errors, but they can also lead to discovery and high-quality care. Second, attendings are well aware that a number of luminous names in academic surgery washed out of their original training programs. In the case of the technically gifted, attendings wish to minimize the type 2 error, that is, dismissing a subordinate as unfit when he is extremely talented. They wish to minimize type 2 errors because they can become a public embarrassment to the department and the judgment of its members, and because qualified trainees who move on to different institutions are important for recruiting future trainees to the program. Third, there is the very real frustration for attendings of seeing a person of talent not fulfilling his potential, despite their best efforts to change this.

In this cohort, resident Josh Carter (whose difficulties with Dr. Arthur were detailed in chapter 2) posed the most difficult promotional problem for attendings. All were agreed on his talent and intelligence. At the same time, all agreed that Carter's work oscillated between the excellent and the lackluster:

> Dr. Pines commented: "I agree with Fred in almost everything he says. This guy is talented and likable. There's no question about it. But I had to jump all up and down on him this spring

to get him to do the work. If he operates, fine, he does a good job managing and observing the patient. But if he's not operating ... [doesn't finish the sentence, just shrugs his shoulders]." Then Dr. Arthur said: "My complaint is that he is unreliable unless he's doing the operating. When you call at night and ask Carter how things are and he says all right, what he means is that the patient he's scheduled to operate on won't die by morning. He doesn't know how the rest of the patients are doing" (Meeting).

The question that attendings had about Carter was, Was his unreliability a part of his character resistant to change, or was it rather a temporary condition caused by his not yet learning the humility appropriate to his station? Carter's experience both in medical school and at Pacific made it difficult to tell which was the case. Attendings reported times when their attempts to discipline Carter were immediately undone by other attendings, who extravagantly praised his work. This process in fact had its concomitant in the promotional meeting as negative statements about Carter were neutralized by positive ones:

Dr. Arthur: "He's great when he's interested. But if he's not, he doesn't give you or the patient the time of day." Dr. White: "I don't know about that, Bill. He worked hard for me and Ollie in September, which was our busiest time. He really stayed on top of things and really pulled a few chestnuts out of the fire." Another attending added: "Look, as I listen I can't escape the feeling that we all know surgeons like this. It seems to be a character type. The question is, do we want to be responsible for training that kind of person? This fellow never rotated through my service, so I don't know him, and I still can't tell from the discussion whether he has a character disorder or whether these problems will go away with maturity" (Meeting).

As the discussion of Carter continued, the attendings' ambivalence about him seemed to grow. He was credited with great talent, intelligence, and the ability to work long and hard hours when motivated to do so. He was damned with being on occasion unreliable, untrustworthy, slovenly, and churlish. Carter's failures, on the whole, were breaches of the standard decorum for care—he violated the rule of "no surprises" too often for attendings to ignore. These breaches of Carter did not always harm patients, but they were seen by attendings as more serious than failures which harmed patients but were rule-governed in terms of medical etiquette. Carter's skills and his shortcomings were so balanced that attendings were unable to come to any sort of decision about his future at the end of the first meeting. They decided to discuss Carter again in their next meeting in a month. The attendings decided to let him know that his future was not yet decided. They hoped that his reaction would give them a clue as to whether he was teachable, or an incorrigible.

In the four weeks that intervened between the first and second meeting, Carter gathered information about what happened at the attendings' meeting. He responded by sending emissaries to those attendings he felt most strongly opposed his retention, and by having extra letters of recommendation entered into his file. These responses angered the attendings and convinced them that Carter's problems were beyond their ability to treat. By mounting what one of his strongest supporters among attendings called a "lousy PR campaign," Carter had missed the point of his critics and proved himself incorrigible. He had shown himself so inattentive to the cues of others that he proved himself unteachable. Further, his response served as evidence that what his harshest critics claimed were his problems—a lack of integrity and a desire to take the easy way out—were true:

> Dr. Arthur said of Carter: "He lacks integrity. What he's done now shows it, and his work with us showed it. To give you an example, one day I asked him if something had been done, and he said it was taken care of. But when I got to the first floor, I found that it hadn't been done. So I asked him what had happened between the sixth floor and the first floor. He answered, 'Well, I gave the nurses orders.' He was probably innocent in the legal sense of the term, but he was guilty of being less than candid. I shudder to think of him as a chief resident." Dr. White said: "As you know, I defended him last month. But the way I feel right now, I don't think he has the maturity to be a chief resident" (Meeting).

After two hours, the attendings convinced themselves that Carter could be made into a competent surgeon but that they were not going to be the ones to take the trouble to do it. Dismissing Carter now, they decided, would serve all their interests best. Another position for him somewhere else could easily be arranged, and he would not be unduly stigmatized for his failure. On the attendings' part, they would be rid of a problem and have more time time for teaching that promised greater returns for their efforts. At the same time, by arranging Carter's placement elsewhere, the attendings at Pacific could continue to monitor his progress and welcome him back into their ranks should he begin to live up to his potential.

There is an irony in Carter's banishment from the medical elite. He was excluded for his inability to meet the expectations superordinates had for trustworthy subordinates. He had failed to properly internalize the norms of the doctor role while displaying great technical talent. Demoting Carter to a training program where the attendings were less professionally imposing than those of Pacific made it even less likely that Carter would accept superordinate authority and hence less likely he would internalize these norms. In addition, it was likely that his considerable technical talents would not develop to their fullest because of restricted clinical exposure. The attendings hoped that, all else having failed, Carter would learn a lesson from his exile from the elite. Given the available options, the punishment fit the crime; however, it was the one most likely to perpetuate it.

Although we have analyzed a cohort of only six, a small sample to be sure, the decisions of the promotion meeting feed back on and lend credibility to the observations of chapters 2, 3, and 4. First, technical and judgmental error is acceptable as long as it can be interpreted as an occasion for learning. However, when made too frequently, such errors discredit a subordinate as a potential surgeon. The commission and concealment of such errors discredit a subordinate as a potential physician entirely. However, the superordinate's ability to control the subordinate are limited. A morally discredited individual in one setting can still obtain license in another. Second, given that subordinates meet technical standards, normative ones become paramount. Those who meet them are embraced; those who do not are rejected. For those who have it, technical proficiency is a rather indifferent indicator of success. Normative compliance with superordinate expectations accounts for who will be retained or fired.[4] Even for those who lack technical proficiency, normative skills determine available alternatives. Attendings themselves are often required to demonstrate that they possess the qualities they demand of subordinates. Their intellectual integrity is displayed in the "hair-shirt" ritual, which models for subordinates the proper way to account for failure.

On Joining the Ranks

Attendings say of the subordinates that they accept into the ranks that "he's our kind of person," or "he's our people." Both phrases end discussion of a subordinate admitted to the ranks of the senior residency. Both phrases serve as a benediction to mark the passage of a subordinate from one whose trustworthiness and skill are always open to question to one who is accepted as a group member.

Besides securing his career for the moment, being certified as their kind of person by attendings has great meaning in the everyday life of the subordinate. When attendings claim that a person is their kind of person, this serves as a preliminary and presumptive moral licensing of that person. This moral licensing has a number of interactional concomitants. Chief among these is a more collegial and respectful treatment of the subordinate by attendings. Once promoted, subordinates are less often the target of attendings' anger and they are less likely to be seen as the responsible agents for culpable failure; as a consequence, they are less likely to be morally discredited.

In the third year of training, the subordinate who makes it that far is relieved of many of the cross-cutting pressures of his role which we saw as responsible for normative and quasi-normative error. The organization of ward work is left to those in the first two years of training. The senior resident is compelled to spend less time at the hospital either performing menial tasks or on call (although his total work hours are still somewhat staggering). He himself becomes dependent on those below him adhering to the rule of "no surprises." When this rule is not followed, the resident joins with the attending in trying to find out why and prevent its recurrence. However, if problems recur, the senior resident can find his attending's approval quickly withdrawn and find himself blamed for not exercising a tight enough control. But as a rule the senior resident is more a junior partner than a servant of the attending.

There are also other subtle changes that occur once one is admitted into the ranks. The third-year resident begins to call the younger attendings by their first names. His relations with older attendings are likely to become cordial, with much more mutual kidding. The third-year resident begins to do more teaching during rounds and ward work. He is allowed to enjoy more of the privileges of rank, and made to suffer less the burdens of initiation.

Admission into senior ranks provisionally admits one to a colleague network. One is seen as a member of the group that has passed the harshest of the initiation rites the profession has to offer. Attendings express this when they say they can "sleep well" knowing a particular resident is in charge. The first two years of training, subordinates are severely tested. For the last three years, they slowly gain acceptance as colleagues.

SIX

Conclusion

Failure to perform competently as a professional means two different things. First, there is failure to apply correctly the body of theoretic knowledge on which professional action rests. Failures of this sort are errors in techniques. For surgeons, we have identified two varieties of this type of error—technical and judgmental. Second, there is failure to follow the code of conduct on which professional action rests. Failures of this sort are moral in nature. Again for surgeons we have identified two varieties of moral failure—normative and quasi-normative. Moral failure is more often the subject of serious social control efforts than errors in techniques. This is to say, social control of the profession subordinates technical performance to moral performance. In conclusion, we shall examine this finding.

First, I shall examine the technical-moral distinction itself to see why moral breaches are considered more serious than technical ones. Then I shall relate type of error to its conspicuousness and to the response it evokes. I shall demonstrate that moral errors are more conspicuous than technical ones and that they arouse a stronger response. A discussion of these relationships informs us how professionals interpret their charter, tells us what license and mandate mean to the professional, and informs us what professionals mean when they claim to exercise professional self-control.

Technical vs. Moral Errors

Embedded in this ethnographic account is the contrast between technical errors, on the one hand, and moral errors, on the other.

Throughout we have seen that moral errors are more harshly treated. At the recurrent everyday level, technical errors are the occasion for restitutive sanctions while moral errors are an occasion for repressive ones. Superiors "support" those that make technical errors and "degrade" those who make moral ones. At the career level those who make technical errors are allowed to remain in the medical elite although they may not become surgeons, while those who make moral errors are banished from elite ranks although they are allowed to become surgeons elsewhere. Why is it that techniques are subordinated to morals? This is not a finding that the literature on professions with its emphasis on increasing specialization and cognitive rationality prepares us for. If anything, as the profession of medicine becomes more scientific, specialized, and bureaucratized, we would expect the opposite. As far as control of performance is concerned, we would expect impersonal evaluations of techniques to have priority over personal judgments of an individual's moral performance. How are we to account for the fact that the opposite is the case?

The explanation lies in the nature of the professional-client relationship. The professional agrees to apply his expertise to the client's problem in a manner that takes care not to abuse and/or exploit the client's helplessness. The professional agrees to protect the client's best interests. The physician does not promise to cure. The lawyer does not promise to win the case. The most that either can promise is to help as best he can and in a fashion consistent with the highest standards of the community. Now, in most professional-client relationships, the client has a great deal at stake. In fact, so much hangs in the balance that suspicion of the professional's motives and the appropriateness of his conduct is always a possibility. To defend against this, the professional proves how secondary his personal considerations are by placing himself in his client's service. He is available when the occasion demands. Moreover, professionals work to cultivate the impression that the only case they have of interest is the one before them now—the client being served at the moment.[1] A professional's claim that he will not benefit from the client's compromised position is backed by the sacrifices of time and energy that he makes for his client. In making these sacrifices, he matches what his client has at stake by a considerable investment of his own.

When things go awry, when the professional's efforts to aid his client fail whatever the reason, the professional's last line of defense—should he doubt himself, should his colleagues question him, should his clients or their representatives accuse him—is that he did everything possible. "Doing everything possible" is a moral defense and not a technical one. The individual claims his conduct is beyond question—that he did everything any other member of his profession might have done in similar circumstances—and that failure is accidental, incidental, and random. He claims that the case deviates so far from the average that it should be discarded from any sample of his normal performance. He argues that its inclusion so skews the sample of his normal work that one might be led to make unwarrantable inferences about his professional worth. The claim that he "did everything possible" is basically a claim to ethical conduct. When he claims that he did everything possible, the professional claims that he acted in good faith. Although results are open to debate, his conduct is not.

The challenges of "good faith behavior" come from three different sources, each at a different level of social organization. First, an individual can doubt himself. Here the claim of "good faith behavior" acts as an individual defense. The individual who convinces himself that he met all the obligations of his office assuages a guilty conscience. Second, a group of colleagues may question an individual's results. This is the professional group exercising its license and mandate. The group standard for what comprises "everything possible" may be stricter or harsher than an individual's. At Pacific the group standard demands sacrifices and imposes on the individual the obligation to recognize problems beyond his level of skill and to route these problems to the proper expert. These last two obligations are meant to assure the widest dispersal of high-quality care. Personal pride or self-interest then does not interfere with the ability to act in a client's interest. The ideal network of professionals is one in which each member in turn is expected to defer to his more knowledgeable colleague in order that skills and problems are properly and speedily aligned. Therefore, the moral behavior of doing everything possible is a guarantee of high-quality technical care. The third challenge of "good faith behavior" comes from outside the profession. Its formal expression is in the legal system. The rules of evidence for what constitutes good faith behavior are established by law rather than being part of an unwritten code. Here we confine ourselves to the professional code in general and to challenges of professionals in the organization specifically. We are concerned with the relation of the group to those members whose action is questioned.

The professional's last line of defense is a moral one because it is proper moral performance alone that substantiates a claim to proper technical performance when events mock such a claim. It is not the patient dying but the patient dying when the doctor on call fails to answer his pages that makes it impossible to sustain a case of acting in the client's interest. It is not losing the suit but losing the suit when representing a plaintiff while having substantial holdings in the defendant's company that mocks a claim of impartial justice. Moral error breaches a professional's contract with his client. He has not acted in good faith. He has done less than he should have. Such conduct is not honest and defensible but undercuts all the presumptions on which the professional-client relationship is based. For this reason moral errors are treated more seriously than technical ones. They undercut the very fabric of client-professional and professional-professional relationships. Hence the control of technical performance is subordinated to the control of moral performance; without the overarching moral system, the technical system is not amenable to control.

Two observations suffice to show the precedence of morals over techniques. First, the claims to excellence made by superordinates at Pacific are based not only on a technical superiority but also a moral superiority. They speak of "sweating blood" for patients or "really busting their butts on this one." The hours they work are a source of complaint but also a source of pride. Attendings feel it is their willingness to do more than their less luminous colleagues which distinguishes them more than anything else. It is this pride in working harder and doing more than others rather than a pride in the advanced medical technology available to them which informs their characterization of Pacific being a better hospital than others. Second, there is the following curious fact. The statistical limit which separates acceptable from unacceptable technical performance has never been firmly established. We do not know how many wound infections make a surgeon incompetent, nor do we know how much undiseased tissue he must remove before his honesty is thrown into question. Here professional standards are not established. Yet the minimum number of moral breaches needed to dismiss a professional from practice is clear-cut: one will do. One breach of professional ethics is all that is necessary to expel a physician from a hospital's staff or disbar a lawyer. In practice, of course, it is rare that a single infraction is so severe as to warrant this response.

The argument should not be pushed too far. We are not claiming that technical performance is unimportant. We are saying that normative, that is, moral, standards are the organizing principle of a professional community. It is worth noting that technical and moral performances are poles of a continuum. In some professions the continuum is quite truncated and any technical error is also a moral one: air-traffic controllers are a good example. In other professions, the continuum is quite long, so long that "not busting your butt" and not doing everything possible—restraining rescuer impulses—can be interpreted as part of proper therapy: psychiatry is a good example. The fact that this is the case allows professionals to accept the occasional technical error even when its consequences for the patient may be grave; defends them psychologically, socially, and legally against charges of exploiting a client's helplessness; and assures the client that his best interests are cared for.

Conspicuous
Performances

The above proof is a rather slender peg on which to hang an argument. We need to demonstrate that the technical control of performance is subordinated to moral controls with stronger data than any we have put forth. In the introduction I claimed that one good reason for studying surgeons in order to investigate social control processes was that their performances were inherently more conspicuous than those of physicians in other specialties. Simply stated, what a surgeon does is more obvious than what a psychiatrist does. We accept as a commonsense assumption that for performance to be labeled "deviant," it has to be somehow observable. Of all medical performances, surgical ones are most observable. After all, it is only these performances that are said to take place in a theater. If our contention is correct that in the concern for social control there is subordination of technical performances to moral ones, we would expect the control of techniques to be a less conspicuous part of the environment than control of morals.

This is, in fact, what we found. Surgeons are loath to judge the technical performance of others. Surgeons routinely condemn results without condemning the performance. They claim that "unless they were there they do not know what kind of situation the surgeon faced, what kinds of factors may have compromised his ability to perform the optimal procedure." They add that "they cannot say for certain what they would have done in the same situation." Because of the multitude of factors that influence judgment and confound results, the social control of techniques remains inconspicuous. When and where it occurs, such control is built into the fabric of everyday life as minidiscussions of surgical problems, as anecdotes or horror stories, as hypothetical questions for future considerations, or as mild rebukes. Individuals are not separated from the work group nor is action seen as in any way "nonnormal" by members of the surgical service.

The fact that controls of techniques are not a conspicuous

feature of group life underscores the problematic and probabilistic nature of medical practice, what Fox (1957a) identifies as the theme of uncertainty in medicine. There are three sources of uncertainty. There are inherent limits to medical knowledge itself; there is the inability of any one physician to master the entire corpus of available knowledge; and there is the difficulty in deciding in any particular case between the limits of the science and the limits of the person. When failure is technical, its source lies in one or some combination of these three sources of uncertainty. To cope with his own uncertainty and to suspend judgment about the failure of others is something practitioners learn early in a medical career. In an unpublished paper on the autopsy as a rite of passage, Fox (1957b) points out that prosectors are careful to specify, in cases where premortem diagnoses do not accord with postmortem findings, the good clinical evidence which informs incorrect diagnosis and treatment. Pathologists are careful not to impugn the motives, skills, or intelligence of the clinician involved.

The point here is that one learns that such a thing as honest errors exist and that all physicians make them. These things happen. There are generally good reasons that one can suggest post hoc for them. It is therefore not proper to damn such results with hindsight. When physicians act in "good faith," the reasons for failure are routinely recoverable and excusable. Moreover, it is assumed that the physician acting in good faith will learn from his failures. There is a general reluctance to let a technical failure be a conspicuous occasion for social control since its sources are so variegated, since the decisions demanded are so subtle and complex, since it happens to everyone, and since it is believed that the responsible physician will draw the proper lessons from the evidence.

While the social control of technical performance is inconspicuous, the control of moral performance is a very conspicuous feature of the environment. With errors of technique, it is never completely clear whether the fault lies in the individual or in the field. However, when the error is a moral one—a case of being improperly oriented to tasks at hand—an individual's liability is quite clear. The social control of moral performance is quite conspicuous. Dedication, hard work, and a proper reverence for role obligations are all readily apparent. A want of interest or enthusiasm in a subordinate is quickly noticed by a superior. From this evidence, superordinates are quick to infer that an underling has serious problems that will interfere with his becoming a high-quality physician. The subordinate's good faith is put into question by his behavior. The judgments that are suspended for errors in technique are not suspended here.

There are three senses in which moral performance and its control are more conspicuous than technical performance and its control. First, subordinates are constantly revealing their moral worth to superiors in a variety of manners: by their degree of attentiveness as they hold retractors,[2] by their affect as they discuss clinical problems, by their rapport with patients, and by their resourcefulness in getting things done. Superiors take all these as indicators of a person's moral performance. Differences in moral performance among subordinates are often greater than differences in technical performance, especially given the restrictions of a strictly regulated division of labor. Moral performance is more conspicuous than technical performance to begin with because superiors find it easier to read a subordinate's moral performance than his technical performance. Deficiencies in moral performance say more about an individual's capacity to improve and become a reliable colleague than do deficiencies in technical performance, which may speak to momentary and easily correctable shortcomings.

The heightened meaningfulness of moral performance over technical performance leads to a second way in which moral performance is highly conspicuous as a basis of social control: namely, moral performance seems more consequential in career-tracking decisions than technical skill. Letters of recommendation or condemnation cite moral character more commonly than mastery of the body of knowledge on which the profession rests.

Despite being talked to several times by Dr. Grant and myself, this man has a tendency to regard the patient as just so much operative experience, and if he is not doing the "cutting and sewing," he is just not interested. He avoids the operating room when he is not going to be the operating surgeon, and takes little interest in cases that he does not find appealing or challenging. In short, he has not performed with the maturity and dependability that one expects of a resident of his maturity in years and apparently this is merely a continuation of past problems.... At this juncture, I just cannot visualize him as a chief resident in surgery as I would be afraid of his slipshod methods and his cavalier attitudes toward responsibility and toward his patients (Department of Surgery).

Letters of praise routinely cite an individual's flexibility, dependability, and sensibility. When asked what they look for in housestaff, attendings cite what they call the three A's: "availability, affability, and ability—in that order." At the promotion meeting, the cutting edge in problematic cases was a person's moral performance. Moral performance governs the sorting of trainees into professional networks. There is a double irony in the fact that technical performance is less conspicuous than moral performance as a basis of social control. One would, of course, assume that moral worth is more difficult to infer from behavior than technical worth rather than vice versa. Is it not believed that, after all, character resides in a more hidden recess of the self than technical skills? Furthermore, the outsider would hardly expect the attention paid to moral performance given the prevailing definitions of the professional as a technical expert who applies a body of theoretic knowledge to perform certain functions valued by the society in general (Parsons 1949, p. 372).

There is a third way in which controls of moral performance are more conspicuous than controls of technical performance. Controls of technical performance are "built into" the everyday performance of tasks. Controls of moral performance are not. They are quite extraordinary disturbances in group life at the recurrent everyday level. They are characterized by the superordinate's assault on guilty parties. Public humiliations and dressing-downs, sarcastic and mock-ironic remarks, or a pointed ignoring of the guilty party are all tactics superiors use to treat moral breaches. This all contrasts sharply with the handling of technical failure, for handling this failure blends into ongoing activity and seems a routine part of it. The manner in which a superordinate handles a moral lapse—his bracketing of the event as something memorable and distasteful—makes these breaches a more conspicuous feature of the environment than technical failures.

Perhaps the greater conspicuousness of moral error relative to technical error is merely an artifact of my research site, which is, after all, a training institution charged with the socialization of recruits. In the world of independent practice, this relationship would not hold up. This objection is an empirical one but empirically I do not have nor did I set out to gather the data to silence the objection. However, I do know that the number of technical errors is much greater than the number of disciplinary actions taken by hospital boards or state medical societies. I suspect that one reason for this is that for error to be considered culpable, technical failure must be wedded to a moral breach. Professionals restrict colleagues—and the extent of this restriction is for our particular purposes beside the point—for abusing the "good faith" requirement of professional action. The restriction of colleagues in other settings—its patterns and extent—is certainly a question for future research. Study of other medical settings and of other professions is of course needed. It would be foolhardy and wrong to argue that my site selection did not limit the generalizability of my data in any way. However, it also provided several advantages, the most important of which was to show professional controls in their most basic forms.

Forgiveness and Punishment

There is a second feature of group life that supports our contention that the control of techniques is subordinated to the control of morals: namely, there is a differential response to these breaches. Superordinates tend to be tolerant and forgiving of technical error and intolerant and unforgiving of moral error. This pattern of response shows us how moral competence acts as the organizing principle of a professional community.

Forgiveness and punishment of breaches are two mechanisms for establishing group membership or the boundaries of the professional group. The first is an inclusion mechanism; the second, one of exclusion. Distinct identity as a group depends on the operation of both mechanisms. If we are to understand the nature of a professional community, we need to look at both mechanisms.

Technical offenses are forgiven by superordinates. This leniency promotes cohesion among members of the work force. Forgiveness itself operates as a deterrence to further technical error. First, it obligates the subordinate who is forgiven to the superordinate who shows him mercy. To repay this obligation, the subordinate becomes more vigilant in the immediate future. Following a technical error, it is quite common for a subordinate to spend extra time with each patient on work rounds double-checking to make sure results are satisfactory. Second, when a subordinate sees his technical errors are forgiven, he recognizes that he has no incentive to hide them. He is less likely, therefore, to compound his problems by attempting to treat problems that are over his head for fear of superordinate reprisal. Forgiveness encourages "help-seeking" behavior and removes the stigma from uncertainty.

Forgiveness also serves to reintegrate offenders into the group. We see this most directly in the "hair-shirt" ritual that is part of the Mortality and Morbidity Conference. The self-criticism, confession, and forgiveness that are all part of this ceremony allow the offender to reenter the group. The "hair-shirt" ritual promotes group solidarity. In tightly knit communal groups such ceremonies are a regular part of group life. For example, forms of this practice are found in monasteries or the rural communes of China. "Hair-shirt" rituals are a form of public exorcism. Through them, whatever demons that led to incorrect practice are driven from the group.

There are parallels in the treatment of errors in technique by superordinates and subordinates. The houseofficer confesses to his attending. The attending confesses to the entire collegium, which is his superordinate. Both humble themselves and in turn both are forgiven and embraced. Forgiveness binds the confessor to the group and exacts a pledge from him to live up to standards in the future. Since in time all make errors in techniques, all are obliged in time to go before the group and humble themselves. Through this process of confession and forgiveness the group exacts the allegiance of all its members to its standards.

By the same token, the group can afford to be merciful in the face of technical error since its members openly confess them. First, such confession is ipso facto proof that an individual adheres to group standards and knows what the expectations for his behavior are. Second, such confessions serve as proof that an individual is punishing himself for his faults. Therefore, forgiveness serves to limit self-criticism and prevent an individual from being immobilized by guilt. Forgiveness helps individuals mobilize for action after failure has stripped them of a sense of mastery. Forgiveness helps individuals cope with the problematic features of medical practice. It is a necessary part of group life which sustains commitments and mobilizes actors in the face of inevitable failure.

Superordinate reaction to moral errors is severe and intolerant. Superordinates punish those who make moral errors. In the short run, they shame these individuals. The degradation of the subordinate who makes a moral error places him outside the group. The onus then falls on the subordinate to show that his lapse was only temporary and not representative of his work. He must show that he "has learned his lesson and been properly put in his place." Those who cannot demonstrate this in the long run are excommunicated from the group of surgeons at Pacific. Demonstrations that one has learned his place are signaled by increased deference to superordinate authority, greater attention to detail, and closer ties with nurses and patients. One makes a highly visible show to the superordinate that one is genuinely repentant.

Superordinate intervention and sanction are necessary for moral lapses but not for technical ones for a simple reason. When technical errors are made, the individual acknowledges his subordination to the group by the gesture of confession and self-criticism. He voluntarily humbles himself. He bows, lowers himself, in the face of group standards. This is not the case for moral errors. As we have seen, the cutting edge that defines moral errors is an individual's failure to acknowledge the underling status which the requirement of "good faith" behavior imposes. The failure to route problems properly because of professional pride or the failure to confess error and admit shortcomings—these are features of moral error but not of technical error. When he makes a moral error, the subordinate shows by his conduct that he does not acknowledge his subordination to the group and its standards. Under such conditions, the superordinate forcefully reminds him of this subordination. The anger that superordinates show on such occasions derives from the manner in which the subordinate has mocked the community and its values.

Just as the group can afford to be merciful in the face of technical error since an individual is contrite, submits himself to group authority, and pledges to do better, the group must be merciless in the face of moral error since an individual is prideful, contemptuous of the group's authority, and offers no assurance of future improvement. The authorities of the group must punish the offender in the second case since there is nothing that suggests the desire or resources for self-improvement. Moral errors disqualify one from civil treatment by the group. Such errors exclude one from the group. One is expected to learn quickly what is forbidden from the fierce response it evokes. Superordinates expect such behavior to be quickly extinguished. When the behavior is not extinguished in the individual, the individual is extinguished in the group.

Forgiveness and punishment are the poles of a continuum on which responses to deviant acts can be arrayed. Discussions of the function of deviance for group formation often emphasize one pole of the continuum to the exclusion of the other. For example, Bensman and Gerver (1963) discuss the importance that forgiving deviance in a factory has for creating group solidarity, while Erikson (1966) discusses the importance of punishment in Puritan New England for maintaining group identity. However, what both studies fail to appreciate fully is that both forgiveness and punishment are different sides of the same coin and that both are necessary if a group is to sustain a distinct identity and boundaries. The proper task of analysis is not to celebrate one process at the expense of the other, but rather to see which violations mobilize one mechanism and which mobilize the other. Forgiveness and punishment always coexist in different proportions in different communities at different times. The task of analysis is to explain these variations.

Corporate vs. Individual Self-Control

We are now in a position to state how professional self-control operates. Professionals forgive errors that are defined as involving techniques. The operations of control for these errors is inconspicuous; it is built into the everyday activities of the work group. Professionals punish errors that are defined as moral. The operation of controls is here quite conspicuous; it is set apart from everyday activities. This is to say that professionals interpret their mandate to control performance as an injunction to maintain a community of high moral standards. Those who show that they are unreliable, incapable of sacrifice, and unable to act in "good faith" in the patient's interest are excluded from the network of elite surgeons and granted only a limited mandate. Those who prove themselves reliable, capable of sacrifice, and able to act in "good faith" are invited into the elite professional network and granted an extensive mandate. In the control of work, technical performance is subordinated to moral performance. Simply stated, physicians do not expect the application of medical knowledge to be perfect. There will always be honest errors. However, physicians do expect perfect compliance with the norms of clinical responsibility. They see this compliance as their best defense and remedy for the honest and inevitable errors they will all occasionally make. Negligence is defined in terms of clinical norms—moral values—and not technical standards.

Unfortunately, we cannot allow matters to rest here. In the term *professional self control*, there is linguistic ambiguity. Read as *professional-self control*, it connotes the individual professional's ability to handle responsibility. It underscores the fact that the client can trust that the professional will restrain his own desire for gain and act in the client's interest. When the emphasis is on the professional-self, the term celebrates the moral stature to which the individual has grown. Read as *professional self-control*, the term underscores the corporate responsibility of the profession to regulate its own internal affairs. This reading emphasizes the contract between the profession and lay society. The ambiguity of the term reflects an underlying ambiguity over the interpretation of license and mandate. We cannot make clear with a hyphen what is an inherently problematic feature of social life.

However, we can point out problems raised by this ambiguity by juxtaposing these two different readings of *professional self control*. From the emphasis in the education of surgeons on character building and the moral development of surgeons, it is clear that the profession places much weight on professional-self control, or the individual's control of his professional self. As superordinates see it, the goal of training is to turn out, after five years, individuals with the capacity to display this professional-self control. We know that education is an imperfect mechanism of social control and that not everyone develops this control. We have seen that those who do not develop these controls are downwardly mobile in professional networks. The question becomes: Who or what controls these individuals as they pursue their careers? What does the corporate control of individual professionals look like when viewed in a setting less exclusive than Pacific Hospital and across settings for the profession as a whole? We do know of the hesitancy of the profession to establish standards which discriminate unacceptable from acceptable performance and of the well-documented tendency (Friedson and Rhea 1972; cf. also chapter 5 above) of the profession to punish by exclusion, thus protecting a few professionals but hardly lay society from less than adequate performance. This suggests to us that there is a hypertrophy of professional-self control and an atrophy of professional self-control.

The hypertrophy of individual self-control and the atrophy of corporate self-control becomes all the more apparent when we focus on the surgery department rather than on the individual service as the unit of analysis, when we look more closely at quasi-normative errors, and when we examine the reactions of the surgeons at Pacific to the "dumps" of their colleagues at other institutions. Analyzing controls on a service, we find a system in which attendings exercise authority without hesitation. Subordinates' errors are discovered and corrected by superordinates. If the error is technical or judgmental, sanctions are restitutive; actions are taken to restore the situation to normal. If the error is normative or quasi-normative, sanctions are repressive; actions are taken which punish the guilty party. In this ritual drama of social control, housestaff and attendings never exchange roles. Superordinates discover breaches and they discover them of subordinates and never of each other. These interactive patterns do not mean that attending surgeons are such moral and technical virtuosos that they never commit breaches which offend the sensibilities of colleagues or even of subordinates. Rather, these patterns speak to the symbolic importance of the completion of training and to the attainment of staff position as a form of moral licensing. Further, such patterns indicate how firmly the norm of autonomy is embedded in medical culture. On a surgical service, professional controls exist in a hierarchical relationship composed of one set of subordinates and two superordinates who are somewhat independent of each other. The domain of social control is limited; each service is a self-consciously isolated unit. The boundaries of the authority system are the scope of each attending's authority. For all intents and purposes these boundaries are never breached. Attending surgeons do not meddle in each other's affairs, unless explicitly asked for advice on a case, or unless making a dramatic gesture of deference to another attending such as first-assisting in a procedure to learn a new technique. At all other times, the respect and freedom which attendings accord each other in organizing their services gives controls their self-consciously isolated quality. Services, then, are the locus of control and not the department. What from one perspective is a detailed and harsh system of controls is, from another, a system in which corporate responsibility is virtually absent and in which individuals are given great license. Within the surgery department at Pacific, quality of care is almost totally dependent on the skills and conscience of individual practitioners and almost independent of any structural constraints save that of hierarchy. Here it is important to remember that a formal hierarchy does not observably govern interaction among attendings on different services the way that it constrains the behavior of individuals on specific services. Individuals on services act within a well-defined hierarchy, while individuals at a departmental level do not. However well behavior is controlled at the service level, at the department level there are no formal devices, save the Mortality and Morbidity Conference, to ensure a uniform quality of care. The Mortality and Morbidity Conference is, of course, a retrospective review of behavior. The surgery department at Pacific, with its highly elaborated conception of autonomy, individual self-control, and its relative absence of corporate controls, is an exquisite miniature of the way medical controls work in general (Freidson 1975).

Rather than merely decry this state of affairs, we are in a position to explain why individual conscience is so well articulated as a control and why corporate devices are so underdeveloped. An understanding of two key mechanisms is crucial here: (1) the attending's authority and (2) quasi-normative error. We have described each service as an independent authority system with the boundaries consisting of the attending's authority. The attending's authority rests on his legal responsibility to the patient. The physician's fiduciary trust is not just a feature of sociological description, it is also embedded within our legal system. So, despite the fact that he makes many of the everyday treatment decisions and that he is responsible for much of the service's operation, the subordinate in a legal sense has no autonomy. He is merely an extension of the attending. When an attending punishes a houseofficer, he is punishing his subordinate as an appendage of himself, as his representative to the patient. In disciplining a houseofficer, the attending is displaying the invisible standards he applies to himself. The superordinate-subordinate relationship permits the dramaturgical depiction of conscience at very little cost to the superordinate. The authority of the attending rests here on his right to care for patients in the manner that he deems proper. This is a power that the house-officer cannot yet claim because he has not yet earned it. He does not have a full professional self. License, the granting of the great personal autonomy, the giving of the right of individuality to the professional himself, is awarded only after training is completed. An attending feels free to reprimand houseofficers as if they were children and often for no better reason than "I'm the boss and that's the way I want things done," for the houseofficer has not passed fully through the sets of rites, rituals, and ordeals that transform outsiders into insiders and make colleagues out of subordinates. But the crucial point is: once such a transformation occurs, a professional self is seen as something inviolable. Cor-porate responsibility is discharged through the socialization and education of recruits. Just as it is inappropriate for parents to meddle in the lives of their grown children, surgeons view med-dling as inappropriate surveillance of the performance of those released from training. In a way, the attending position on social control may be characterized as follows: For the five years they are home—while they are housestaff—you work hard with them, you try to provide a good environment, you send them out and you hope for the best. The corporate responsibility of the profes-sion is not seen to extend beyond raising one generation of sur-geons after another from professional infancy to professional adulthood.

However, as in any socialization period that takes a substantial portion of time, the relations among the generations is marked by conflict. Quasi-normative errors as a symbolization of this ine-quality among the generations allow us to understand this conflict more fully. A complete professional self is one that has earned the right to organize its work in a manner that it sees fit. This right belongs to attendings; it does not yet belong to house-

officers, although they often claim it. Quasi-normative errors act
on two distinct levels as boundary-maintaining devices that uphold the privileges of rank for attendings. First, such idiosyncratic standards of proper practice establish the right of the
attendings on each service to employ their own best judgment in
carrying out their work. What it is "wrong" for housestaff to do
on one service, an attending on another service may do as a matter of standard procedure. The judgment, maturity, honesty, and
suitability for a surgical career of a houseofficer who makes
repeated quasi-normative errors would be open to question. Yet
attending A and attending B view the differences between themselves as nothing more than an artifact of training, clinical experience, individual philosophy, personality—in a word, as a
difference in style. In this setting, differences of style among
colleagues are recognized as legitimate. To reduce many matters
of disagreement about proper practice to questions of style removes them as a serious topic for discussion, or possibly control.
For while one may like or dislike a style, one very rarely finds in a
style cause for moral outrage and social control. That large area
surgeons relegate to style when evaluating one another (and error
when judging subordinates) serves to underscore their autonomy
as professionals while diminishing the range of practices seen as
open to public debate and control. Quasi-normative errors—that
is, the stylistic idiosyncracies of attendings—serve to isolate the
surgical services from one another.

Second, and perhaps in the long run more significant, is the
way quasi-normative error serves as a device to maintain the
boundary between attending and housestaff. The attending has
the power to impose his will on a situation whatever the merits of
the arguments a houseofficer may muster to defend his course of
action. At an everyday level, events treated as matters of style
among colleagues are treated as matters of morals between ranks.
The fact that attendings react in a similar fashion to normative
errors, where there is consensus within the collegium, and also
react similarly to quasi-normative errors where there is no consensus, may have several regrettable consequences. It may mean, in
the first place, that the moral lessons of normative error have not

been properly internalized. Housestaff mistakenly link similarities of response to similarities of stimulus and confuse genuine norms with quasi-norms. They treat all repressive sanction as flowing from the arbitrary, capricious, dogmatic, and unreasonably autocratic personalities of attendings rather than from deeply held common sentiments shared by a community of fellow surgeons. In this case, they would be unable to develop strong commitments to the community norms since they would be unable to perceive that such norms exist. All shortcomings become attributable to personality and style. In the second place, the treatment of quasi-normative error cultivates in housestaff an appreciation for the pains of subordination. The completion of training signifies being out from under. The houseofficer, in talking about the future of a prospective surgeon, emphasizes his freedom to make his own decisions, his freedom from others' eccentricities, and his freedom from the opinions of others. Here, quasi-normative error weakens a future surgeon's ties to a colleague community and at the same time fails to instill a finely etched sense of what constitutes good and bad practice. Independence, freedom, and professional autonomy become completely egoistic; the ritual passage of residency can fail to transmit the culture to the recruit. Furthermore, quasi-normative error serves as a gloss for attendings to lean on the authority of their office rather than their expertise. Labeling a behavior a quasi-normative error closes off discussion of its appropriateness without an assessment of its merits. Such labeling prevents the give-and-take necessary to keep attendings sharp. Finally, quasi-normative error can depress housestaff initiative and zeal and thereby encourage the mindless following of routines.

The behavior of the surgeons at Pacific to the "dumps" of colleagues elsewhere is yet another indicator of how undeveloped corporate responsibility is within the profession. "Dumps" are mismanaged patients sent to Pacific from other hospitals. Basically, surgeons do not publicly condemn or reprimand the most outrageous performances. Their rationale is twofold: (1) if the surgeon is a responsible, ethical colleague, he knows he has made a hash out of the case, so there is, as the surgeons say, "no reason to rub his nose in it"; or, alternatively, if he is not responsible and ethically competent, then the dumping surgeon is a "bandit" and nothing anyone says will change him; and (2) either way one has it, if one complains and makes "dumping" unpleasant and difficult for the surgeon in trouble, he would rather bury his problems before suffering the "bad manners" of Pacific staff and seeking help for them. Silence, then, is seen as the response that best protects patients. At Pacific, the response of superordinates to "dumps" is to crack the whip harder over the heads of their subordinates in the hope that negligence is a generational problem and that their redoubled efforts to establish professional-self controls, a well-articulated sense of individual responsibility, will eradicate such lackadaisical behaviors. All the while, the attendings at Pacific fail to instill such controls in some subordinates and release them from training—and from their watchful eyes—to send dumps to Pacific in the future. The problem is not, as some have claimed (Barber et al. 1973; Gray 1975; Crane 1975) an absence of any socialization, controls, or ethical sense in the profession; the problem is rather a system which celebrates individual conscience as a control while ignoring corporate responsibility. The profession of medicine needs to develop structural remedies—or structure socialization—in a way that brings into balance both the corporate and the individual dimensions of control. Adequate controls in the profession exist only to the degree that a corporate moral sense is cultivated equal to the individual moral sense.

Summing Up

In this report we have described the system of controls that regulates behavior among surgeons. We have discovered what these controls are, how they are enforced, how they have far-reaching consequences for channeling fledgling surgeons into different career paths, and how these standards are learned by subordinates. We have seen why the controls which do obtain in the profession are so uneven. Being matters of conscience, they may be very strongly internalized by individuals or they may be only weakly present.

The findings of this report differ from those of others in ways that should be made clear. First, Freidson (1970) and others who follow him emphasize the hesitation with which controls operate and the mildness of most punishments. The position of those who emphasize "professional dominance" give sociological credence to Shaw's famous dictum that "all professions are conspiracies against the laity." We have found, however, that these patterns cannot be explained adequately as maneuvers by the profession to retain a stranglehold on the market. What we have found is that the hesitation and mildness which surrounds controls are best understood in light of the way a surgeon's knowledge about the world is structured. The uncertainty which the surgeon routinely faces in making a diagnosis and pinpointing a precise causative agent for therapeutic misadventure accounts for a great deal when explaining why surgeons discipline errant colleagues as they do and when explaining why normative rather than technical breaches are the more serious errors. In short, in understanding social control in a profession I feel it is best not to stray too far from the cognitive frameworks the profession itself employs to make sense of the world. To take the role of the other impels us to look at how the other constructs his world. We need to know which objects in this world are taken for granted, which are problematic, and which are considered irrelevant for the purposes at hand. If, in the study of lower-class deviance, it is unwarrantable to bootleg everyday definitions of right and wrong into our work, it is just as inadmissable to do so in the case of high-status professionals. One of the strengths of this report, not common in other works in the field, is that it attempts to take the sociology of knowledge of modern medicine seriously, the better to see how the nature of a particular cognitive realm structures values, attitudes, and practice with regard to error. A sophisticated sociology of medicine must have some familiarity with, at the very least, the nature of medical reasoning in order to appreciate the coded language in which colleagues raise questions, communicate approval, shoulder blame, and hurl accusations at each other. I am not saying that all studies in the sociology of medicine should necessarily display this understanding of the physician's phenomenal world; I am saying only that we need to place a greater emphasis on such understanding in the future than we have in the past. As sociologists, it is peculiar that we have such appreciation for the "symbolic" interaction and linguistic codes of corner boys, prostitutes, drug users, fences, members of communes, and so on, and so little appreciation of and tolerance for the same dimensions of action among physicians.

The recent work of Barber, Crane, and Gray claims that physicians receive almost no ethical training through their socialization. My claim is that postgraduate training of surgeons is above all things an ethical training. Subordinates are harshly disciplined when they violate the ethical standards of the discipline. They are promoted and accepted into the ranks as colleagues on the basis of their ethical fitness. It is true that the moral standards demanded and the superordinate's self-interest converge here to a great degree. Nevertheless, the point remains that normative standards of dedication, interest, and thoroughness are applied in evaluating subordinates rather than narrowly technical standards. Moreover, ethical dilemmas such as how to most appropriately manage the terminal patient are discussed during rounds. The moral and ethical dimensions of training are not bracketed from all other concerns but are instead built into everyday clinical life. It is unwarrantable to infer from absence of formal courses, seminars, and so on that ethical "training" is relegated merely to the informal structure of role learning. Perhaps one of the reasons that Barber, Crane, and Gray missed the ethical dimension of training is that their survey research methodology is too distant from the rhythms of everyday life to capture this dimension of action. Time and again surgeons express their feelings by indirection—the horror story is a good example. To understand how surgeons debate ethical concerns requires knowledge of that same coded language surgeons use to discuss error. I am not suggesting that sociological analysis is a subtle, new form of mysticism which requires a divining of the real meaning lurking beneath the surface of interaction. On the contrary, I suggest that sociological analysis begins with an understanding of what actors mean when they talk to each other. Such knowledge requires a respect for the word and gesture as units of social meaning, a respect that rests on our understanding of the *gestalt* which structures any word's meaning. Since we expect each occupation to have a unique *gestalt* based on its typical work problems, we expect members of occupational groups to speak to each other in their own coded ways. To learn the language of an occupational group, to learn its ways, we need to spend time observing how they meet the routine contingencies of the workplace.

Once we learn the ways workers speak to each other in the workplace, we see things that were previously obscure. A third difference in this report from others concerns the nature of in-group solidarity among professionals. We commonly believe that physicians maintain a conspiracy of silence, protecting incompetent colleagues by shielding their mistakes from the lay public. This account makes clear that this silence is not merely a feature of professional-client relations, but that it is also a feature of the public confessional, the Mortality and Morbidity Conference. When an attending "puts on the hair shirt," he takes blanket responsibility for a case. He maintains a conspiracy of silence. He does not publicly announce which subordinates made which errors. The in-group solidarity of the service as a working group would be crushed by such an open betrayal of its confidences. In a sense, Mortality and Morbidity Conferences such as Pacific's serve as a model of the lesson "we don't tell tales" as well as "we openly admit our mistakes and strive to correct them." Conspiracies of silence are not in and of themselves evil things. They are, however, harmful when they allow a group to practice without any incentives to curb their excesses. A problem exists for the profession of medicine when the lessons of silence are learned without the concomitant lesson that the professional himself has the responsibility to correct his errors. Professional responsibility is itself thought of as individual and not corporate responsibility.

This last point leads me to make a concluding recommendation. I feel that improved performance is desirable, necessary and possible in the social control of medicine. Such performance rests on the profession's developing a corporate sense equal to its individual sense. While it is impossible to specify, in a step-by-step fashion, a program for accomplishing this, my account makes clear what elements contribute to an effective control system. First, there must be some hierarchy, or a functional equivalent, that permits question-answer sequences, what we call the competence quizzes of rounds, about the appropriateness of different treatment modalities. Second, some face-to-face interaction is necessary. Physicians need to feel part of the same community and answerable to one another. Third, there must be public forums for discussing problems and allocating blame. Such forums create as well as sustain a community by giving members a sense of their shared identity. Fourth, the community needs some control of sanctions so that it is able to control malefactors within its own ranks. The dilemmas involved in handling "dumps," or in dismissing subordinates from Pacific only to lose the capacity to restrain them, need resolution. At present, a physician's conscience is not only his guide but the patient's only protection. The patient deserves the protection of not only the individual's but also the collectivity's conscience. Beyond that, the profession as a whole needs to raise its conscience about its public responsibilities. The collectivity needs to promote the structural changes that will build stronger accounting mechanisms into everyday practice.

Appendix

The Field-Worker and
the Surgeon

All fieldwork done by a single field-worker invites the question, Why should we believe it? It would be nice to be able to claim that I was a totally impartial observer whose characteristic ways of looking at the world allow an almost perfect mirroring of some objective reality. However, as the fieldwork experience made clear to me, I am not without my biases. I would like to pretend that this was not so for any number of reasons, but the observer role in some sense trained me to see these biases in a heightened way. As I reflect on the experience of eighteen months of participant observation in a teaching hospital, and on the dilemmas of the observer role, I feel a sense of respect for data-collecting procedures which allow the researcher to keep the sensuous world at a distance, and which thereby allow him to avoid the self-exposure, self-reflection, and self-doubt endemic to field-workers. In the field, the everyday life of his subjects overwhelms the researcher, threatens to obliterate his sense of self, and forces a reconsideration of deeply held personal and intellectual beliefs. It would be of little point, then, for me to pretend in the face of such a powerful experience that I was merely a coding machine which transcribed the events of everyday life first into field material and then into the sociological and literary order of the preceding pages. In this appendix, I would like to describe the field experience itself and the analysis of the data. This appendix should show the reader how I identified and controlled for my own biases and should allow him to control for them independently of me.

In the Field

How did I begin? The first thing I did was to approach an attending I had met at a party, explain my proposed study, and ask for his cooperation. The attending expressed enthusiasm for the project, but refused his cooperation. He claimed that if I wanted to really be trusted, I would need the housestaff's acceptance. He expressed his fear that his sponsorship would be a "kiss of death": housestaff would view me as his spy and never talk freely with me. If I wanted my project to succeed, he advised, I needed to be seen as my own person. So rather than somehow magically start the research, he gave me the names of a number of residents and the hospital's central page number. What I learned during this interview was that there was no instant access for the field-worker. Not sure if I was receiving aid or a runaround from my initial contact, I called the first name on his list, the chief resident. We met for coffee and I explained my plans. The resident approved my being an observer on his service, but claimed he would have to check with both attendings. The chairman of my department provided a letter of introduction to the chairman of the Department of Surgery. Gaining my initial entrée was a multistaged diplomatic problem. Each interaction was a test, and access was the result of continual testing and retesting. Entrée was not something negotiated once and then over and done with. I was always entering new scenes and situations involving different combinations of people. Fortunately, of course, I could rely on what I had learned in previous encounters and the repertoire of roles that I had developed and that others developed for me. The important thing that field-workers must keep in mind is that entrée is not a single event but a continuous process.

Access—being allowed in the scene—is one thing, but approval and trust of field subjects is quite another. Just like access, cooperation cannot be ordered by fiat, but is rather earned again and again, when the field-worker shows that he or she is trustworthy and reliable. Much is made in fieldwork accounts of the "cover story" which the observer uses to explain his presence in the setting as a first and essential step in gaining trust. My cover story was very simple. I explained that I was doing a dissertation on the way surgeons learned to recognize and control error. The surgeons were, as a rule, remarkably uncurious about my research. None ever questioned the legitimacy of my research question or the nature of my methods during our initial meetings. Few even requested that I account for my presence. I was not asked for my cover story very often and, when asked for the story, I was not required to elaborate on it. In some sense, my access was secured by sponsorship of housestaff trusted by all. Once my access was established, my cover story was superfluous and served as a gloss during introductions. In the everyday course of things, my housestaff sponsor was more important to my access than any cover story I used.

Trust was gained neither during initial introductions nor by the artful manipulation of a cover story, but through my performance in roles I assumed and was assigned by housestaff and attendings. Housestaff assigned me a number of roles. Most generally, I was an "extra pair of hands," and a "gofer." During the time of my fieldwork, I became very proficient at opening packages of bandages, retrieving charts, and fetching items from the supply room. Through these tasks, I expressed some solidarity with whatever group I was observing and gave something, however inconsequential, in exchange for "observing rights." Second, I was an "emissary from the outside world." My round of life was less circumscribed than a houseofficer's: I read and watched more news, saw more movies, and participated more fully in university life outside the hospital. In some sense, I provided housestaff contact with a world they felt cut off from. During Watergate, I always brought a number of papers into the hospital. How or why this became my task I do not know. Often I purchased these papers at the hospital gift stand, a place interns and residents certainly had access to. Their general reluctance to pick such papers up is not so much a mark of their frugality as a symbolic statement about their relation to the world outside Pacific Hospital. I later learned that housestaff attach a magical property to newspapers, books, and magazines. If they bring them in to work they see this as jinxing themselves and condemning the group to an impossible busy day. It is, however, permissible for outsiders to bring such taboo items to them. My passing remarks about movies, current events, the weather—all were taken as an indication of what educated people on the outside were thinking. Third, I was a "fellow-sufferer." As a graduate student not released from training, I was perceived as occupying a position analagous to the houseofficer's. My own career problems and expectations were topics that houseofficers initiated much conversation about. They constantly compared and contrasted our different experiences. During such exchanges, houseofficers constantly emphasized the indignity of their roles and often suggested that their present burdens justified their future rewards. From me, they sought to learn about the generalized indignities of the subordinate role in sociological training. I regaled them with my wildest recollections of coding data and proofreading galleys.

Fourth, I was a convenient "sounding board." I was surprised at the degree that informants sought me out to relate stories of practice that they disagreed with. Feelings that were not shared in the group, discontents, uncertainties were taken to me. I knew that observers were often sought by organizational malcontents; what surprised me was that all my informants were at one time or another malcontents. Such a label was not a stable organizational identity as much as a fleeting reaction to behavior, which for one reason or another offended the houseofficer's sensibilities. Disfiguring palliative operations, patient discomfort, and the openness of communications among the ranks were the most common complaints. As a "sounding board," I was implicitly asked to play a quasi-therapeutic role: to listen without judging and to understand. The fact that I was asked to play this role so often by so many speaks both to their understanding of what an observer does and to the deep feelings that physicians repress as a matter of course. As a rule, we, as medical sociologists, have not concentrated enough on how fragile physician defenses are, what events disturb them, and how primal the existential material they are dealing with is. Birth, life, death are not questions that one works through definitively. We need to pay more attention to the provisional nature of the resolution physicians make to the conflicts such subjects present. My own graduate students in the field now report that their informants ask them to play this quasi-therapeutic role, also. Like me, they find it both disturbing and flattering. The fact that our subjects choose to use us in this way suggests both that we need to learn methods for containing and managing these encounters, and also that we cannot define the field-worker role totally in instrumental terms. We come to have identities for our subjects quite independent of the ones we promote for ourselves. Ironically, it is often these identities that yield the greatest amount of data.

Fifth, houseofficers viewed me as a "referee" in conflicts among themselves over patient management, quarrels over the equity of the division of labor, and disputes about whether or not patients understood what was happening. In the midst of such disagreements, one houseofficer would turn to me and ask: "Well, what do you think? Which of us is right?" These were not comfortable situations for me when I could hide behind the observer role. A judgment was demanded as the price for my continued presence. Moreover, any judgment was certain to alienate one of my informants. I developed tactics for throwing the question back to the disputants or for pointing out the merits of either side, or making a joke of the entire dispute. Over time, I tried in vain to teach my subjects that such conflict resolution was not a proper part of my role. Nevertheless, being asked to referee disputes was a recurrent and always problematic task and not one that I ever felt totally comfortable with. As I felt more accepted, I was somewhat better able to put questions off. But in the beginning, I was stiff, uncomfortable, and always mindful of my relationships with each party. As a referee, I was able to elicit good material when I was able to turn the dispute into an occasion for discussing different attitudes and beliefs toward medical practice. Unfortunately, I was not always levelheaded enough to accomplish this because I felt so put-on-the-spot by such confrontations.

Sixth, I was the group "historian." Because of the way housestaff rotate through the various services, it was not unusual for me to have been on either the Able or the Baker Service longer than any particular houseofficer. When this occurred, I was expected to know something of the history of the different patients on the service. I was expected to keep track of attendings' remarks and verify them for absent group members. The role of group historian served me well, since it forced housestaff to depend on me for information that they needed. This created a greater sense of mutual obligation between housestaff and myself and to the degree that the information I supplied was reliable, I established my credibility. Also, I was a short-run as well as long-run historian. I would often ask housestaff about action that I could not watch but was interested in. (Much work is done individually, and on any given day I saw only a portion of possible action.) On more than one occasion, my questioning reminded houseofficers of a task that had until then slipped their minds. My unwitting reminders saved them from oversights which would have gotten them into trouble. The fact that such incidents occurred further indebted housestaff to me and heightened my legitimacy. A fieldworker pays a price for this kind of legitimacy, though. The historian role itself presents some of the most common moral dilemmas that a field-worker faces. Each time I gave such a reminder to a houseofficer, I changed what would have otherwise happened without this intervention. Lab tests, consultations with other physicians, and conferences with patients and their families—all these were on occasion events that took place because I reminded houseofficers of them. By jogging the memory of houseofficers in this way, I made it impossible for myself to observe what happens when these events fail to occur. On these occasions, I did not intend to alter the natural course of events; but it did happen that I unwittingly created an occasional participant-observer effect.

Despite the fact that it was not my intention in these instances to change the action I was studying, one can see very clearly that errors of omission present the observer with a moral dilemma. If one does remind a houseofficer, one disturbs by that act the very relationships one is attempting to study. However, if one does not remind the houseofficer—and yet knows he has overlooked something—it is possible that a patient's care will be compromised. On most cases when I asked if something had been done, I did so because as a sociologist I was particularly interested in seeing or hearing a report of that specific action, and usually because I was unaware of whether it had occurred or not—I was trying to orient myself. If the houseofficer had forgotten about the task I was asking about, if it had completely slipped his mind, then that fact told me something about the difference between a sociological perspective and a surgical one; and I learned something more about the structure of the surgeon's life-world. There was one category of event, however—conferences with patients and families—that I asked about more than others. Here I was often conscious of my participation in the scene, but thought that some patients (exactly which patients these were and why I reacted to them the way I did is a complex matter that I do not understand) deserved fuller explanations than they often got from the surgeons. A question that I cannot answer is, Did the surgeons see my role as a sociologist such that they presumed that I was interested in such group phenomena, and did they come to rely on me to remind them of their diffuse obligations to patients and their families? Is this the major role they assigned me in the group? If it was, who was responsible for making sure that this team responsibility was filled when there was no sociologist present? Whatever the answers to these questions, a rule of thumb I applied was to keep my reminders as few as possible. This was a rule I occasionally broke because of my feelings for a patient and his/her family. I must also confess to one other category of event on which I routinely broke my own rule. As a group historian, I occasionally asked questions that served as reminders to subjects that I felt were hostile and/or skeptical of my sociological enterprise to establish that I belonged in the field; that I was concerned, aware and helpful; and that I was a legitimate member of the group. The fact is I occasionally used my questions to demonstrate the ways the group needed me. (One could also argue at the same time I was proving to myself that I served some useful purpose in the group.)

If errors of omission present observers with one type of moral dilemma, errors of commission present him with another. In the case where the field-worker knows that some harm has been done to a patient through physician or nursing error, does the observer have any direct, ethical obligations to the patient and his/her family? That is, should the field-worker either inform the patient or find some alternative means of making public the error? I chose not to do this for a variety of reasons. As a pragmatic matter, being a patient-advocate would have made the kind of fieldwork I wanted to do impossible. Moreover, I felt a responsibility to other medical sociologists who wished to undertake field projects in the future. I was aware that my conduct could either make the way more or less difficult for those who followed me. While some participant-observer effects seem acceptable to me, others, those that contravene the basic operating norms of a group, are not acceptable. These larger effects not only distort the phenomenon under study, they make it impossible for later field-workers to gain access to and legitimacy within medical settings. Most important, I felt I could discharge my ethical obligations to patients more effectively by describing the general categorization and management of error rather than tilting at windmills in one or two select cases. On the face of it, this kind of advocacy would not seem to be much of a problem; in fact, it is hard to imagine a field-worker, insistent on imposing his definitions of justice on a scene, completing his work. However, this fact is not as significant as the importance of recognizing the strong feelings that observing in a hospital evokes, and restraining the "rescuer" impulses that witnessing so much pain, suffering, and death provokes. Whatever roles houseofficers cast me in or I assumed, the major irony of the field-worker role was always apparent: on the one hand, I was intimately involved in all aspects of the everyday life of a group; and on the other hand, I was constrained by the nature of my task to exert as little social influence in that group as possible. So, my sensitivity to the group's actions and their consequences was heightened at the same time that my theoretic commitments restrained me from even raising the group's consciousness about the effects of its own actions.

I had less intimate contact with attendings than with house-staff, and assumed and was assigned a narrower range of roles. Most commonly, I was seen as any other "medical student." Attendings assimilated me to the group by treating me like any

other member of the group. They had me look down proctoscopy
tubes, rake abdomens feeling for a mass, and learn to hold
retractors properly. Their treatment of me helped strengthen my
ties to houseofficers, who saw that not only was I not in league
with attendings, but that, like them, I was the occasional butt of
an attending's sense of humor. By the same token, my own
willingness to take part this way in group life served notice to
attendings that I was willing to do what was necessary to complete
my project. When attendings viewed me as a medical student,
they often tried to teach me concise medical lessons. Whatever
problems of identification and rapport I might have had, it is
interesting to note that attendings had some of their own. Toward
the end of my fieldwork, two attendings approached me, told me
that I must be interested in medicine to have spent so much time
at Pacific, and then informed me that if I wanted to go to medical
school, they would help me in any way they could. I took their
offer as an indication that perhaps I had been in the field long
enough.

The incident above is related to another role attendings cast me
in—their "advisee." Attendings offered two types of advice. First,
there was "scientific" advice. Here attendings would address
themselves to the design of my study. They wanted to know about
my control groups, my measurement instruments, my hypotheses, and all similar paraphernalia from the type of research they
engaged in. When I would explain that my model for research
was somewhat different than theirs, they were skeptical but generally tolerant. After all, I was the sociology department's
problem, and not theirs. Second, attendings offered "interpretive
advice." When we were alone, they would often explain why they
acted in certain situations the way they did, what they felt to be
the burdens of their authority, what the major problems doing
surgery in a major medical center were, what the personal
strengths and weaknesses of their colleagues were, and so on.
Like houseofficers (although the opportunity arose less frequently), attendings unloaded themselves on me. It is worth
noting here that I was ten years younger than the youngest

attending, so the fact that they used me as a "sounding board" points to ways in which the surgeon's role remains disturbing even to those who have practiced it all of their adult lives.

In addition, attendings used me often as a "clown" to diffuse tensions in the group. When things were going poorly, attendings on occasion would question me like any other member of the group and then poke fun at my fumbling and ignorance. Sitting around the doctors' lounge, the rigors of academic life would be compared unfavorably with those of surgery; and my manly virtues would be impugned. It was not always as a clown that attendings used me to ease tensions. Just as with housestaff, I was asked to referee conflict. My study was used by them to deflect conversations from their course. So that often when faced with troublesome questions from nurses or other physicians, they would give a noncommittal response and then ask me to explain my study. They would ply me with questions until they were sure the conversation could safely resume. These three roles were not assumed with equal frequency nor were all assumed from the first day of fieldwork. From the beginning and most generally, I was assimilated as a medical student. Then I was used as a "diffuser of tensions." If I passed the test implied in this role, I became an occasional confidant of the attending. With one attending who was not greatly invested in clinical issues, I was never other than a quasi-medical student. With the others, I played all three roles, albeit with varying frequency and intensity.

So far in this description I have concentrated on the various roles I played in the field setting. The rationale for this is simple. In the analysis of our fieldwork data, we concentrate on the role relations among participants in the scene we choose to study. Yet we often pay comparatively less attention to our own role relations with the subjects who make our knowledge of the setting and of the action possible. Since in fieldwork these relationships are our major methodological tool, they require serious discussion. How we manage these relationships determines the depth, validity, and reliability of the data we collect and the inferences we draw from it. We need devices that ensure control of our like and dislike of various participants, the weighting that we give

incidents, and the ways our own everyday roles impinge on and
create strains with the field-worker role. The problem of objective
description and analysis is in itself formidable even if one were
only observing a television program, for example. In fieldwork,
the problem is made more complex because of the deep relationships and attachments one builds over time to one's subjects. As
Charles Lidz (1977) has correctly pointed out, the right and
privilege of being an observer is a gift presented to the researcher
by his host and subjects. So the observer has, in addition to
whatever the other problems that becloud his structured role-
relations with his subjects, the very special problems that attend
the giving and receiving of gifts. I would agree with Lidz that the
recognition and proper understanding of the gift relationship
serves as both a convenient theoretical framework for understanding the peculiar dilemmas of the field-worker and at the
same time a formidable restraint on bias in observation and
interpretation.

First, what are the special features of the gift relationship? As
Mauss (1967) pointed out in his classic statement, the giver and
the recipient of a gift are involved in an interactional sequence
that involves giving, receiving, and reciprocating. Even more
important, involvement in a gift cycle creates a solidarity among
participants and signifies that they have obligations toward each
other that extend into the future. The fact that the field-worker is
both the receiver of a gift and a guest means that he has a diffuse
sense of obligation to his host-giver-subject. Field-workers have
long recognized their indebtedness to their subjects. In fact, as
one reads accounts of fieldwork itself one senses that this burden
is truly "the magnificient obsession" of those who employ this
research method. While not explicitly analyzing the observer role
as a gift relationship, field-workers worry, in their writings, over
fulfilling their obligations to their subjects, over balancing personal debts to individuals against universal debts to the discipline
of sociology, and over discharging obligations to subjects that
extend beyond the life of any particular piece of research. In
addition, there is the field-worker's typical ethical dilemma: what
if the data I gather are potentially harmful to my subjects? What

if the facts themselves betray those to whom I have become so attached over so many months? Others have spoken of the "tyranny of the gift" in different contexts, but it is clear that the gift of access, of witnessing social life as it is lived in someone else's environment, exercises a tyranny of its own. This tyranny has as its most distinctive features three significant elements: (1) the danger of overrapport, so thoroughly merging with the subject's point of view that one cannot achieve the critical distance necessary for analysis; (2) the danger of overindebtedness, so thoroughly feeling a sense of diffuse obligation that one can no longer assess what one does and does not properly owe his subjects; and (3) the danger of overgeneralization, so thoroughly idealizing one's subjects that one sees their behavior as overly representative of all persons in a class.

I was protected from overrapport and overindebtedness in part by the very structure of hospital life. Unlike field-workers who spend years with an unchanging population, my subjects rotated through the surgical services fairly rapidly. Some stayed for as little as a month; none stayed over three months. There were housestaff I liked very much; housestaff I detested; and others I barely got to know. Whatever the case, there was an unending parade of housestaff. The mere fact that I was observing so many people in rapid succession prevented overrapport with any one subject. There was, of course, the danger that I would identify with the structural position of being a houseofficer, even if I avoided strong attachments to specific individuals. After all, I was a twenty-four-year-old graduate student, subordinate to a dissertation committee, and struggling to achieve autonomy within my own profession. Surely there was a clear and ever-present danger that, being a subordinate myself, I would overidentify with the subordinate and his problems. Overrapport with housestaff was avoided by two features of my everyday life. First, my wife, Marjorie Waxman, was supervising child-care workers in a psychiatric hospital at the time of this research. My conversations with her made me sensitive to the problems of the superordinate, especially the difficulty of balancing the needs of patient care with the needs of subordinates to develop their own skills and judgments through their own mistakes. Second, my major field-supervisor constantly pointed out to me instances when I seemed to take subordinate complaints too much to heart and urged me to see beyond the specific perturbations in housestaff-attending relations to see what are generic problems in superordinate-subordinate relations. Of course, I also had to guard against the opposite problem, overidentification with attendings. After all, did they not have, to an exaggerated degree, the autonomy I was working so hard to obtain? Here, I was protected from over-rapport by a number of factors. First, my relations with attendings were not as regular, intense, or relaxed as those with housestaff. Second, several of my own friends in medical training served as constant reminders of the subordinate's problem. Third, there is a general resistance in sociology to sympathize with the perspective of authority. Authors such as Becker (1970) constantly remind us whose side we should be on.

My resolution to the problem of overindebtedness was somewhat different than the resolution to overrapport, and unfolded over time in two quite separate phases. A moderately sensitive observer of life in the surgery wards of a hospital will be flooded with feelings of helplessness. These feelings themselves have two distinct components. First, witnessing so much pain and suffering, the field-worker wants to roll up his sleeves and do something, anything. At the same time, seeing death as an everyday event makes one guilty and overly aware of one's own good fortune. As a field-worker, I was often made uncomfortable by what I saw. I felt I had stumbled into incredibly intimate and significant slices of patients' and doctors' lives. Much like any person who sees more than he would like of a friend's life, I felt guilty about some of the knowledge I had gained, worried over what the boundary between privileged information and data was, and wondered about how I repaid my obligation to my subjects. In the short run, the housestaff resolved the problem of helplessness and indebtedness by the roles they cast for me. When housestaff demanded that I help out by wheeling the chart rack, opening dressings, acting as a group memory, they provided me a means to cope with my own helplessness and assuage my guilt at the same time that they incorporated me into the group. While I was in the field, my involvement in the group resolved for me the problems I experienced as an indebted guest.

These problems reemerged when I left the field and began writing up the report. I saw much that was wrong in surgery, but what I saw emerged against the background of dedicated people working tirelessly at very difficult and complex tasks. What if what I reported was harmful to those that made the account possible? I had the problems of balancing my universal obligations to sociological analysis to my particular obligations to my research subjects. Unfortunately for me, I could not expect anyone to point the way by the everyday roles they cast me in. One thing I did was not begin writing immediately on leaving the field. Before drafting this report, I let the freshness of the experience recede somewhat so that I would not be overwhelmed by the memory of my relations with particular individuals. Second, when recording field notes, I made every attempt to keep my description of events as behavioral as possible, and my recording of conversations as verbatim as possible. At all times, I tried to keep "in situ" analysis separate from my field descriptions. I kept two different categories of field notes: (1) a log of happenings, conversations, and conferences; and (2) a separate running analysis. In this way I was later able to identify for and correct problems that resulted from overreport or over-indebtedness. By this procedure, I would see where the data confirmed, or failed to support, my analyses. There is in fieldwork always the problem of selective data collecting and analysis that might harm one's subjects. Any definitive resolution to this problem awaits more sophisticated, but at the same time unobtrusive, techniques of gathering field data. At the present, the length of time we spend in the field and our own intellectual integrity is our only protection to this problem. Third, I shared my report with the surgeons upon its completion. We discussed areas of disagreement between our interpretations. In particular, they objected to the rhetoric of sociology; they saw my framing the problem with a deviance and social-control vocabulary as unnecessarily pejorative, but they accepted (even if they did not agree with or fully understand) my rationale. They agreed that I had most of the phenomenological description right, if not always the interpretations. However, where there were interpretive disagreements, the surgeons attributed them to my being a sociologist, and accepted my analysis as valid from my frame of reference. They suggested ways that I could better protect the anonymity and confidentiality of individuals. For example, at their request, I changed the pseudonyms I originally chose and excised all dates from my field materials. I resolved part of my debt by allowing the surgeons to observe me as a sociologist at work.

Overgeneralization is also a recurrent problem for field-workers at two levels. First, there is the danger that one particular event will become etched in the field-worker's memory as emblematic of the way action is organized in an environment. That is to say, field-workers may overgeneralize incidents and see them as representative of categories of action. Second, field-workers may overgeneralize from their particular sites to all other types of similar settings. In the first case, I avoided overgeneralization by making sure I had at least two independently generated examples of the same phenomenon before I began to make inferences. My operating rule here was, as far as I can see, not fundamentally different than those that survey researchers use to ensure reliability in their studies. Also, I was very careful to follow particular incidents through many levels of social organization. For example, I was able to test my inferences about normative error in the promotion meeting, where I observed the criteria attending surgeons use to judge the fitness of housestaff for surgical careers. Throughout my fieldwork, I was very careful to test observations in one context against those of another. On the other hand, there are observations I made that did not find their way into the fieldwork because I felt my inferential base was too thin. On one occasion I watched a series of unexpected deaths and complications, which occurred in quick succession, temporarily destroy the morale of Able Service. These occurred during the end of a rotation, while a chief resident was on vacation. I developed an explanation which related the occurrence of failure and group panic. However, during the rest of my fieldwork, I did not have the opportunity to observe another rash of failures. As a result, such speculations did not find their way into the manuscript. As an aid to the reader, I have tried to indicate throughout the text where inferences are based on slim observation.

There is a second type of overgeneralization—generalization from the specific case, Pacific Hospital, to hospitals that are not included in Pacific's class. Pacific is a member of the medical elite. There are perhaps twenty hospitals in this country with the same reputation for excellence that Pacific has. I am confident that the description of controls at Pacific is one that fits virtually all members of this class. I am also confident that I have described and analyzed a professional "ideal type," an environment where the major preoccupations have to do with the aesthetics and elegance of surgery, uncontaminated by such mundane matters as fees, social networks to generate referrals, and market pressures. How the system of social control I described is modified in more modal settings is a question that deserves further research, as is the question of how comparable it is to the systems of social control in other professions. These are questions that I am beginning to work on now. There is certainly no intrinsic reason that fieldwork cannot be as cumulative as any other area of sociology. The benefit of using a site like Pacific as a starting point is that physicians there are quite self-conscious about their place in the medical world, and make explicit reference to why they deserve an esteemed place in the profession. Moreover, being so self-conscious, they are eager to inculcate into their young recruits the values in which they believe so strongly. Attending surgeons see their trainees as extensions of themselves in many ways; one of these is that they expect the conduct of those whom they train to reflect honor and glory back on Pacific.

Out of the Field

One peculiarity of field research is that one discovers what one learns in the field often only after one has left the field. So, strangely, the most creative and fruitful periods of field research are those where the researcher steps back from his immersion in an alien world, takes stock, and decides where to go next. By alternating periods of total immersion with periods of analysis, the field-worker can avoid phenomenological fatigue, that is, the sense of "I've seen it all before," and can continually refine and sharpen the questions asked of a particular research. For this study, I normally spent two or three months in the field, full-time, recording my observations in as straightforward a manner as possible, left the field for two weeks to a month to analyze my data, and then returned with a greater sense of what I now knew and what I still had to learn about the conduct of surgeons. For example, after retreating from the field the first time, I discovered in my notes that surgeons treated some mistakes as normal occurrences, while other events were treated as quite extraordinary and unacceptable performances. But at that time, I did not know why one set of events was categorized by actors in one way and another was so differently treated. It was clear very early in the study that the seriousness of an error was not determined by a set of precedent variables such as the patient's age or social status, nor was it determined by such antecedent variables as what happens to the patient. An error's seriousness was related only incidentally to the patient and his condition. On the other hand, seriousness was related in a very direct fashion to the attending's reaction. Discovering this, I felt reassured and at the same time I knew nothing, since I did not know what determined the attending's reaction.

My first immersion in the field in some sense determined the direction of most of my subsequent observation, as I tried to unravel what the bases of attending evaluation were, how clear these were to housestaff, and how widely they were shared among all members of the team. A dialectic of immersion and reflection that began the first day I arrived on the surgery wards at Pacific— and which I am sure is not completed—allowed me a continuous sense of discovery. It is worth noting, for instance, that I did not discover quasi-normative errors until after I left the field entirely. I had not seen while in the field so clearly how the lines of cleavage among the ranks were structured. In turn, my new understanding that there were two distinct types of normative error forced me to revise my conclusions about the social controls in surgical training by allowing me to see some of the ways its ethical content is undermined. I also gained a new respect for what it means "to let your field data speak to you." There are any number of things about the field that one discovers only by not being there. I discovered the "charisma" of surgery, not in the hospital but at parties and other social events. Being a sociologist does not normally make one the center of attention; however, being a sociologist who studies surgeons does. As my research progressed, I was struck by the almost primal awe my friends and acquaintances had for surgeons. Normally sophisticated urban dwellers with Simmel's (1970) blasé attitude would literally beg for details about what surgeons were really like, about what went on in operating rooms, about what their doctors were really like. It occurred to me that I had, through my close association with them, borrowed part of the surgeons' charisma. Seeing that the surgeons' charisma was not just some dramaturgic creation in organized social settings helped me understand how the surgeons' autonomy was as great and unchecked as it was. It also made me see that this was not simply a result of surgeons' behavior but was also nurtured by patients' needs and desires. Cocktail party curiosity also alerted me to how little people know about the medical care they receive, how few people have ever been in an operating room as an observer, and how powerful and coexistent are the contradictory impulses both to glorify and to degrade the surgeon. (Cocktail parties also taught me of the need for circumspection and tact, which I shall comment on below.)

Unfortunately, I did not learn as much from leaving the field as I might have, because I did not keep a careful record of why I chose to leave the field at the times I did. I assume that had I been as clear as I might about my comings and goings, about what was going on in the field that would make me willing or eager to leave, then I might have gained some greater understanding than I have about the surgeon's life space. I know there were days when I had to force myself to go to the hospital, and other days when I grabbed at any straw as an excuse for a breather. But when and why these feelings intensified at the times they did, I do not know. Such knowledge is of more than private psychodynamic interest (though it is of that also), for it helps make clear what strains field-workers are subject to in medical settings, how they can better prepare themselves, and how they can be better supervised. The end result from such understanding would be more valid and reliable monographs, less likely to be subject to any "observer effect."

Data, Confidentiality,
and the Field-Worker

I indicated above that I learned some lessons at cocktail parties about circumspection. In a literal sense, this is not true; but social situations presented me with a sticky problem. When I was in the middle of the field, disguising the place and principals of my study was not as easy as it is in this report. I was always aware when I spoke that others knew those I spoke of, and that a too-loose tongue could hurt me and them in many untold ways. Since I promised my subjects confidentiality and anonymity, the "cover story" I devised to manage social situations was as consequential as the one I devised to manage field introductions. Only by assuring confidentiality and anonymity could I satisfy my subjects that my study would be within the bounds of current medical ethics. Both promises present some dilemmas, however.

First, I could not ever be sure that some enterprising person would not be able to figure out my place and principals. Essentially, confidentiality and anonymity were the promises I made but I had little control over their fulfillment. There have been recent debates about whether field-workers should go to the bother of making general "covering names" for their sites, and whether they should disguise their subjects. It seems to me that such fictitious names do more than provide confidentiality and anonymity: they highlight the generalized features of our descriptions and minimize the particularized aspects. To my mind, this aspect of naming is even more important in some ways than confidentiality and anonymity in that it creates a fieldwork literature rather than a description of specific places; for example, Bellevue, Long Island Jewish Hospital, Johns Hopkins.

Others have advocated that to make fieldwork more rigorous and to display our methodology more openly, we should open our notebooks to the curious. Such procedure would allow others to see how we manipulate our data and fit the canons of science in general. Such a proposal troubles me because, as a sociologist, I gathered litigable material from subjects who trusted me. As a sociologist, I have no legal right to claim a privileged or confidential relationship with my subjects; my notes are subpoenable. If I opened my notebooks in the manner necessary to make clear the operations I performed on my data, I risk having those notebooks put to uses other than those I approve of by people whose motives I may distrust for reasons I think are less than just. Involved here is a difficult problem: how to afford my subjects and myself enough protection so that we feel comfortable doing the study, at the same time displaying my data in a way that assures others of the validity and reliability of my research. I have indicated for the reader what I have done to satisfy myself of this report's accuracy. For the moment, I suggest that this—along with giving and receiving adequate supervision—is the best I can do.

Conclusion

As a research method, fieldwork yields results that often are phenomenologically rich, theoretically provocative, and practically useful. The major liability with this research method is that there are no procedures internal to the techniques of field research itself that control validity and reliability. The major datagathering technique that the researcher utilizes is his relationship with his subjects. For better or worse the rules that govern relationships are less precise, harder to articulate, and more complexly interwoven with other normative systems than the rules that govern, for example, item construction on a questionnaire. By the same token, the field-worker's sampling procedures and

the manipulations he performs on his data are often left unex-
plained. Clearly it is not that field-workers do not gather data by
rules, sample from everyday life in a complex fashion, or manipulate their data. Rather, it is the case that to state what the rules are
requires statements of such generality that they are of little use
in any particular setting. The reason for this is not hard to understand: our subjects are never simply subjects. They also occupy a
variety of other roles and the rules that govern relationships, for
example, with physicians are different than those that govern
relationships with heroin addicts. This inherent variation imposes
on the field-worker his special obligation. The field-worker must
describe the role relations that he had with his subjects as clearly
and honestly as he can. The field-worker must describe how he
avoided overinvolvement or on what occasions he succumbed to
it, how he avoided overgeneralizing, and how he avoided overindebtedness to his subjects. A clear statement of the social
matrix out of which the field materials emerged allows the reader
to judge validity and reliability for himself. At the same time, it
has the added benefit of providing comparable accounts of the
fieldwork experience which allows us to see what is general to a
researcher's relations to his subject and what is particularly his
own.

An Amended Appendix

An Ethnographer's Apology, a Bioethicist's Lament—The Surgeon and the Sociologist Revisited

After rereading his novella, *A River Runs Through It*, Norman Mac-Lean said that he would not change so much as a comma. Having read that work, I agree. Beyond that, I envy MacLean his certainty. After periodically rereading my own work, there is much that I would change. I remember that just before *Forgive and Remember* was published I obsessed about the possibility that I got this or that detail wrong. I then went on to magnify my obsessions: What if none of the interpretation was correct? What if I used my data to construct a plausible delusional system? I knew that I had written a tight, coherent argument. But I also knew that nothing is so coherent as the ranting of a paranoid. I was not particularly reassured by the kind words from my informants who looked at the manuscript and commented on how much I had gotten right. In fact, such appreciative comments merely fueled my panic. I had not created an independent delusion of a specialized social world; I was not that creative. What I had done was more pedestrian; I had simply bought into and crudely represented the surgeons' collectively organized and professionally shared delusional system. Irrational as they were, such were my fears on the eve of publication.

I had always been taught that a good fieldwork account contained insights unpleasant to subjects, the dirty professional secrets that subjects would prefer to keep hidden, the ass end of the sacred. There was, I also had been taught, a similarity in fieldwork and psycho-analysis—both make the latent manifest—the truth of what is brought to light is indexed by the amount of resistance these new insights provoke. The implication of these beliefs for me, as an ethnographer, was that if my subjects approved of what I had written, if they identified with it, if they liked it, then I must not have penetrated too deeply into their world. And so it went. On the eve of publication, I still went back and forth between two conflicting fears. Either I made it all up or I just stated the obvious. In the end, I comforted myself with the thought that though veracity was a goal, though a commitment to getting the facts right was what separated ethnography from fiction, I still had told a good story, a useful story. I began to think that maybe what was important was not literal or even interpretative truth, which I now saw as an elusive goal. What was important was to create a version of reality that would in Levi-Strauss' memorable formula be "good to think with."

With this conviction, I suppose I could claim some sort of foresight. I was a post-modernist ahead of the curve. I would gladly claim credit if I could. But the conviction that a good story was the best that I could do felt much more like a face-saving rationalization than an epistemological belief. In any case, as an empirical sociologist, I saw a clear difference between believing that many interpretations of one reality were possible and believing that only multiple interpretations existed, none more authoritative than any other. The fact that in surgery people acted and as a consequence people lived or died, professional actions were judged, residents and nurses were most likely to be found wanting, predisposed me to the "someone here has the power and authority to make decisions that matter" model of social life. The voice of unchallenged organizational authority in *Forgive and Remember* is, as the epilogue makes clear, the attending surgeon. I never directly challenged the authority of the attending surgeons in everyday decision making—it would have been the end of my study. I gave voice in the text to the residents' complaints, but constantly reminded the reader how unrewarding frontal assaults on authority are for floor nurses and residents. The grumblings that I give voice to were all expressed in settings and at times when attending surgeons were not present.

Even so, it is more than twenty years later, and I still find myself bothered not by the story I told but by two stories I chose not to tell. At the time, each of the two omissions that I am now about to remedy struck me as not just morally justifiable but as morally necessary. But with all the hindsight that a long stretch of time provides, I see that each omission had theoretical consequences for the story I told. Each blunted the interpretation, analysis, and critique of surgical training and professional socialization, shop-floor ethics, and professional social control embedded in the ethnographic account.

The first omission occurs in chapter five, "Climbing the Pyramid: Professional Control and Moral Identity." The chapter is an attempt to show how attending surgeons' everyday judgments of residents' performance exert a career influence. The chapter is described as a natural experiment testing the book's major hypothesis: namely that technical and judgmental errors were blameless while normative and quasi-normative errors were blameworthy. The chapter unfolds to show how this is the logic attendings use either to promote residents to the next level of training or to deny such promotion. The chapter "demonstrate[s] that the promotion decision is a presumptive moral licensing that provisionally admits or blackballs a subordinate from the fraternity of academic surgeons" (149).

In the chapter, only the behavior of residents is problematic. I do not stop to question whether the criteria, standards, rationalizations, or processes that attending surgeons employ might themselves be problematic. I also do not display any of the data that I collected that would allow others to raise these questions. The absence of such data is important. Ethnography is less good to think with if it does not provide a rich enough database to allow readers to frame alternatives, to disagree with authorial certainty, to see things differently. Here I am documenting how omissions made *Forgive and Remember* less good to think with. I edited my data, changed a critical fact (and I recognize that changing the facts contravenes some rather stringent ethical norms of science) and, in so doing, made my own work less rich. I did so in order to obey the canons, as I understood them, of ethnographic ethics.[1] What is offered here is offered in the spirit of correction and apology.

1. To speak of this under a rubric as ancient and formulaic as canons of ethics is a misrepresentation in the extreme of how I thought about the omissions at the time. I did not think about these omissions in a way as systematic and organized as invoking canons of ethics suggests. At the time, each omission seemed reasonable and necessary—as time has passed, and as we shall read in but a moment, I now think one of the omissions was justifiable and the other not.

This then is an act self-revision; as such, it is not clear how much of this should be done in public. There is a thin line between improvement and indulgence. I tread it in the hope that, on balance, that the discussion presented here falls on the positive side of the ledger.

Changing the Facts

I suppose the time has come to present what was initially misrepresented, to correct what was changed. In order to make the correction I need to present a large section of text. The following material describes the promotion meeting at which surgical faculty meet to decide the fate of second-year surgical residents:

> The faculty agreed as quickly as they did in Smith's case that a second candidate, Jones, lacked the technical skills necessary for a surgical career. But in this second case, they had grave doubts about whether Jones had any place in the medical profession at all. Jones combined technical maladroitness with an inability to admit mistakes and difficulties in communicating with patients and staff. This had led on occasion to small correctable errors growing into catastrophes.
>
> > Dr. Gray opened discussion of Jones by reporting: "Jones has had a lot of problems over the last fifteen months. This morning I talked with him and told him that an inability to communicate with peers and patients was not a quality we were looking for in our residents. I suggested to him that he meet with Dr. Cantor in psychiatry to discuss whatever personal problems he has before he makes any plans to continue his career in any capacity. He was quite adamant that he needed no help and that he wanted to be a surgeon." Dr. Grant said: "I did not know what to make of Dr. Jones his first few days on our service, but I have reluctantly come to the conclusion that this man is sick. I don't trust him around my patients." An attending asked, "How do you mean sick—physically or mentally?" Dr. Arthur answered, "Mentally. He's off his rocker. Totally out to lunch. He needs help and he needs it quick. The question is not whether we should keep him, but whether he should finish out the year. In my

mind, I wonder if he's on drugs." Dr. Gray then said: "As I
said before when I gave him the option of seeing Dr. Cantor,
he was totally opposed to it." Dr. Grant added: "There is no
doubt he needs help. Yesterday in clinic he was really around
the bend. He couldn't focus on patients. You could not have
a conversation with him. He couldn't deal with anything."
Dr. Peters commented that "it doesn't sound like much has
changed over the course of a year. Maybe he has a brain tumor." Dr. Ross said: "If he has a problem, I don't think we
could in good conscience let him go without offering him
help. I think we have a responsibility to see that he gets
proper care. But our responsibility to our patients comes
first. If there is any doubt about his stability, we cannot continue to let him see patients." Dr. Gray then summarized the
comments about Jones by saying: "Then we are all agreed.
Not only will Jones not be offered a position, but he will not
be allowed to return to duty until he is investigated by someone in neuropsychiatry" ([Surgery Department Faculty]
Meeting).

The attendings felt some responsibility for Jones as a person
under their care. However, Jones' breaches were so consistent
and so consistently denied by Jones that immediate expulsion
was necessary. Unlike Smith, Jones was not a tracking problem.
He was a total problem that attendings wished to rid themselves
of entirely by shifting responsibility to the psychiatry department.
     The contrast between the handling of Smith and Jones sup-
ports my argument about the differences between technical and
normative error and also suggests inherent limits to professional control (156–57).

What the analysis nowhere suggests is that those inherent limits have
to do with biases in applying available standards to mete out appropriate sanctions. In the above, I refer to Jones as a gendered person ("him,
he, his, this man") a total of thirty-four times in the space of one manuscript page. All of these references are deliberately misleading; Jones
was the sole female in the cohort of surgical residents I observed.
     When drafting the manuscript, I did not think twice about changing

Jones' gender. I had promised my subjects confidentiality and anonymity. There was no way that I could think of to keep Jones a woman and honor that pledge.[2] So "she" became "he," and the analysis proceeded without missing a beat—a study of standards and their use. I raised no questions about whether those standards that reinforce group norms and that are so transparently fair on their face are ever used in ways that reinforce existing prejudices and inequities. The fact that I shared the attendings' discomfort with Jones, as did virtually all of her peers, helped blind me to the impact of gender. Jones was difficult to talk to; among the residents she was the one who avoided me the most and who volunteered the least. And what she did volunteer, I often had difficulty understanding. Beyond that, if Jones did distrust me—and I always sensed that she did—for me that was further proof of her limitations. After all, I was different than the male attendings and residents. I knew that, and I was not yet wise enough to see why Jones might quite reasonably not know it as well. I never gathered data that dealt squarely with how Jones understood the effect of her gender on her career as a surgical resident. Jones was silent with me and I did not know how to break through that silence. As a result, I never gave voice to her complaints, never allowed her voice to challenge directly the authoritative voice of attending authority.

I'd like to be able to say that today, anonymity and confidentiality be damned, I'd never change gender again. I recognize now that it is too important a determinant of behavior to ignore. Unfortunately, this is a goal that is hard to uphold. Before the publication of *All God's Mistakes*, one of the genetic counselors complained that her identity was too thinly veiled (I had kept gender and ethnicity correct when assigning a pseudonym). She wanted her name changed to "Bill Smith." I fussed and fumed but I did what she asked. I did not think I had any

---

2. Years later, when I first discussed this gender switch with colleagues, one asked, "Why not keep Jones a woman and make another resident one as well?" I thought it a good question with a ready answer. The question itself was a sign of how times had changed. The fact that that alternative never occurred to me says something about the gender composition of surgical training programs at the time of my fieldwork. I did not think about this option because the notion of two women in such a small program strained credulity.

choice. I had promised her confidentiality and anonymity and I felt I had to do anything she felt necessary to assure them, even if I thought the request unreasonable. But the two instances differ—in one case, a subject asked for protection; in the other, I provided it without being asked. In a peculiar way, the change involving Jones offered more protection to the surgeons of Pacific Hospital than it did to Jones. I don't know if Jones felt protected or if she desired anonymity. In fact, for the longest time, I didn't know what became of Jones. After the faculty meeting at which it was decided that she have coercive psychotherapy before resuming her duties, I never saw her again. Neither did anyone else. Faculty and residents alike knew only that she had moved out of her apartment. No one knew where she was. She had disappeared without out a trace, as powerful an indicator of her social isolation within the group as one could imagine. When I first had the idea of for this second edition, I decided to interview Jones and Carter to see how they viewed the events that *Forgive and Remember* chronicles. I knew where to find Carter and I set about to track down Jones. What I found on the internet was a recent obituary that indicated that Jones had risen to great prominence in the world of emergency medicine. This confirmed that there was something amiss both in the original assessment of her performance and my unquestioning acceptance of it.

So now, over twenty years later, I look at the text and wonder how I could have left gender out. A good many of the points feminists make about male domination are present in the brief vignette: Dr. Jones is placed in the sick role and seen as a candidate for psychiatric care (She's "totally out to lunch," "around the bend"). One physician even suggests, somewhat illogically since there had been no progression of symptoms, that "maybe she has a tumor." Another suggests that Dr. Jones is "on drugs." At this point in the 1970s, she would not have been alone among the surgical residents at Pacific if she engaged in sporadic, episodic recreational drug use. Who knows—perhaps that activity would have had the beneficial effect of connecting her with her peers in a mutually shared activity.

I have no doubt that changing genders theoretically impoverished my discussion of the moral order of surgical training. I also have no doubt that under the circumstances I had little choice but to switch Jones' gender. As a result, no matter how alive to the nuances of gender

I might have been, no matter how alive I was to why Jones had so much trouble communicating (and I was not as aware as I think I should have been), I was not free to share this knowledge with readers. In the text of *Forgive and Remember*, I go on at great length describing how much informal communication and bonding goes on in the surgeons' locker room and the attached lounge. I detail in the text how the atmosphere of the locker room assuages and blurs for a time the hierarchy of an academic surgical service. In the locker room, surgeons relax, war stories are shared, and group solidarity is reinforced. Such moments were not planned; they did not happen according to a schedule or every time surgeons changed from street clothes into surgical greens. In fact, what is magical and wondrous about such moments, what intensifies the shared intimacy, is their randomness. They are not in any ordinary way planned for or predicted but they do happen. Predictable or not, such moments were not shared by Jones. She dressed with the nurses. She never hung around in the male lounge. Jones may have been unable to communicate because she did not get many opportunities. Beyond that, I realize now that without doubt Jones worked in a "hostile environment" and that she was a victim of sexual harassment. (I will explicate my reasons for this below when I deal with the second omission in *Forgive and Remember*.)

In multiple ways, I was more a member of the team than Jones: I shared a locker room with the guys, played squash with them, slept in the same on-call room (Jones had a separate room), drank beer with them, shared lewd comments about the nurses, and swapped smutty stories. I was one of the boys and Jones was not. Here it is perhaps important to note that Jones and I were often misidentified by those who did not know our actual social identities. A sociologist in white lab coat and surgical greens, I was often thought to be a surgical resident. A surgical resident in lab coat and scrubs, Jones was often thought to be a nurse.

On those occasions when I have discussed with others my discomfort now about switching Jones' identity then, I have been told that I am being unnecessarily hard on myself. I am judging my behavior by standards that did not apply at the time. While I think this is largely true, it is cold comfort and it points to a larger problem. Whenever I ask myself: how is ethnography justified as other than a privileged and self-

indulgent professional activity? and what should ethnography do?—
part of my answer is always ethnography provides data with which to
critique the in between our actions and our ideals. If we are trapped in
the values of the everyday, how do we do this effectively? Beyond that,
when we alter our data to protect our subjects, how do we know that the
data we alter is not critical? What is an innocent change and what is
not? (Davis 1991 and Chambers 1999). My problem with changing
Jones' gender is that it makes the critique I did not make impossible for
others to make. To say that I was a prisoner of my times seems too convenient, too exculpatory. After all, it was not as if there were no critiques in the late 1970s of the patriarchal excesses of medicine. It
seems to me that what happened was more complex—a conflict with
one sort of value (anonymity and confidentiality) led me to betray, wit-
tingly and unwittingly, another kind of value (commitment to an egalitarian society).

The Second Omission

Above I suggested that I was sure that Jones was a victim of sexual harassment because she worked in a "hostile environment. This is a serious charge and I do not make it lightly. Yet there is very little in the text
that would support such a charge. I do indicate that the work of being a
surgical resident is stressful. But I generally paint a picture that has that
stress flowing quite naturally out of the intrinsic problems of doing
surgery at a major academic medical center—difficult cases that lesser
surgeons will not touch, the shortage of ancillary services that routinely plagues academic medical centers, and the violent trauma and
tragedy that are all too common in the inner city.

There was a dimension to the stress that I quite consciously chose
not to mention. That dimension was the hectoring, often abusive behavior of senior surgeons. One of the reasons that I am so sure that
Jones was sexually harassed is that verbal harassment was a rather routine event for all residents, regardless of their gender. Senior surgeons,
many of whom had their first experience as battlefield surgeons, believed that residency was a stress test. Part of surgical training for them
was recreating the battlefield conditions they felt were so critical in developing their own excellence. So when the world did not throw

enough problems in the fledgling surgeon's way, then the senior surgeons occasionally felt free to create some on their own.[3] The most
spectacular incident of a "private stress test" that I observed did not
find its way into the text of *Forgive and Remember*. Before I explain,
let me describe.

I have been sifting through old field notes for more than a few hours
over a couple of days now. While this unexpected stroll has had rewards all its own, the time-stained foolscap that I had been seeking has
eluded me. This baffled me. There were more field notes in manila
folders than I remember writing, each recording encounters that I had
long ago forgotten. Yet missing were notes I recall writing that described an incident I recall as if it had happened yesterday. But the
notes describing the particular incident that I wish to present are
nowhere to be found among all the other notes that so meticulously describe people, places, and incidents that I no longer remember witnessing.[4] I am about to describe, in single-spaced indented form to

3. To be fair, there was a great deal of variation here. Some senior surgeons never harassed, embarrassed, abused, bullied, or treated their residents with disrespect. Other senior surgeons rarely missed the opportunity. If that formulation is too strong, then
perhaps it is more accurate to say that very little inhibited their attack impulses. It is
worth noting that the more mild-mannered surgeon often had nothing but contempt for
his, and now sometimes her, more histrionic peers. Whatever feelings the theatrical attending created among his colleagues, they suffered in silence. I never heard one senior
surgeon correct or confront another. But, then, this is probably not the kind of activity in
which two senior surgeons would engage in front of the novice outsider.

Additionally, I suppose, one might argue that *Forgive and Remember* was written a
long time ago and that surgeons no longer behave in any of these ways. The abusive behavior I am about to describe no longer takes place. That I think is true. But, then again,
I chose not to include the incident that I am about to describe because it was so unrepresentative. However I recently have had occasion to interview all faculty and residents in
six neurosurgical training programs. Reports of the total demise of the dramatically hectoring surgeon are exaggerated.

4. The very fact that the notes describe so much that I have forgotten seems strange to
me. When I was doing the fieldwork, recording the notes certainly felt like a needless
chore, a species of academic ritualism—"how could I ever forget this?" I thought. Going
back over the forgotten notes somehow vindicated the importuning of my teachers at the
time and justifies my current nagging of students in the field. The notes themselves index
a peculiar feature of fieldwork—we collect so much data and present so little of it.

signal typographically that it is from field notes, an incident which occurred over a quarter of century ago but which is being written up in
the present. In texture and detail, the note is a pallid copy of the lost
original. I suppose this takes me from the realm of revision to the realm
of creation. Empirically what I report here is an ethnographic urban
legend that can't be verified. Anyway, here is something that happened
that I can not find in my notes; something, in other words, that I have no
business reporting as data:

> I am late and not for the first time. I change alone in the locker
> room. As I change, I muse. I just have a white lab coat with ad-
> hesive tape covering its rightful owner's name. I do not have a
> hospital I.D. card. I have been at this fieldwork over a year. How
> come I have never been stopped as I move to and from re-
> stricted areas of the hospital alone—SICU, patient rooms, X-
> ray, supply closets, nurses' stations, doctors' lounges, E.R.
> treatment rooms, the O.R.? Once as I bolted from a toilet stall
> where I was taking notes and raced from the latrine without
> flushing or washing my hands, I was dressed down by an at-
> tending and given a lecture on proper hygiene. But, of course
> the very fact that he felt free to lecture me indicated that he
> never doubted that I belonged to one of Pacific Hospital's train-
> ing programs. I suppose that early in the fieldwork I thought it
> necessary to take notes in a toilet stall indicated that I was not
> so confident that I legitimately belonged at Pacific as the attend-
> ing who chastised me was. What kind of security system is it
> that can be breached by race and gender alone?[5] I wondered,

5. To be truthful, I know that the lost note that I am reconstructing here did not have
these musings about hospital security, which has considerably tightened in the wake of
baby snatchings and assaults on hospital personnel and patients. Other notes, however,
that I did not get to work into *Forgive and Remember*, do contain these musings and the
toilet stall incident did actually occur on another day early in the fieldwork.

As an index of how things have changed since I did the fieldwork on surgeons, consider the following: I never received any formal administrative clearance to do the research for *Forgive and Remember*, had no consent form, and never really though much
of the ethics of proceeding without formal consent. When after reading the publication
contract for Forgive and Remember, which held me liable for any legal actions consequent to publication, I suggested to my editor that the hospital attorney review the man-

how did the attendings, so intolerant of the residents' lateness, view mine?

I raced into the operating room feeling, as always, slightly ridiculous in a green scrub suit, the bottoms of which I can never tie properly, paper booties, hairnet over a massive frizz, hastily tied mask, and fogged glasses. I enter operating room three looking for the Baker Team. They are in room two, I'm told. I enter room two from the scrub area. Dr Arthur greeted me with effusive sarcasm. Sarcasm itself was not unexpected, his taking special notice of my presence was. "Oh, good, the sociologist has joined us. How nice of you to come, Bosk." He was hanging on the side, unscrubbed—The Homeless Surgeon—this too was unusual. Christian was performing the surgery. Carter was acting as his first assistant.

After a short pause, Dr. Arthur spoke to me again, "Have you done your Mother's Day shopping yet? Perhaps Dr. Christian [who is German]could make you a lampshade from the cuttings and trimmings today? You know, Christian, I haven't seen this much blood since your relatives greeted the chief rabbi of Berlin during the war."[6] Arthur went on like this for a while. After he failed to get a reaction from Christian or Carter or me (we are both Jewish), he moved on to others. He turned to the anesthesiologist (who is an Asian woman) and, invoking his experience as a field surgeon during the Korean War, made some derogatory comments about "slopes, gooks, and dinks." When Arthur failed to get more than a roll of the eyes from the anes-

---

uscript, the attorney was surprised that the research had been done but not unhappy with the result.

Of course, clearance and consent, as I later found out, are not much of a protection—for the researcher at least. (In truth, they are not intended to protect the researcher.) I had both for *All God's Mistakes* (Bosk 1992). Nonetheless my physician-subjects tried to block publication and threatened a lawsuit. In this second case, the hospital attorney was less surprised and less delighted by the appearance of a manuscript (for a fuller description see Bosk 2001).

6. In the previous note, I indicated that the "reconstructed" note above contained materials that I was certain were not in the original. Here I should add that I am certain that these words were spoken in just this way. Much as I have tried to forget, to repress, these words, I have never had much success. But without the original note, you'll just have to take my word for it.

thesiologist, he turned to his regular scrub nurse (who is black) and asked her, "Do you know how many times I had to practice this operation on blacks before they let me do it on whites?" The scrub nurse did not respond. Instead, she asked Christian if he was ready for some instrument or suture material. Failing to get a reaction, Arthur began to grumble about the pace of the surgery, then fell silent, and left the room as his residents prepared to close.

After the surgery was completed, after evening rounds were completed, I gathered with the residents in the cafeteria for dinner. Josh Carter was fuming: "I couldn't believe Arthur today. Did you ever see a bigger Jackass? I felt like slugging him." Christian said: "It's part of his making everything a stress test. You have to let it go in one ear and out the other." Carter then turned to me: "I'm not like Christian. I can't stand that shit. But it's part of what we have to put up with if we want to get through this program. We have to shut up and take stuff like that. Look I'm Jewish and so are you, I don't know how you felt but I felt like walking out of the operating room. I don't really want to scrub with him anymore. I don't know if I can take it. But what choice do I have. If I say anything, I'm gone. So you have to shut up and take it. But did you ever see a bigger shithead than Arthur today?"

Truth was I probably had not. Arthur was a complex character, insulting one day, charming the next. With Arthur, one never quite knew what to expect. One did know that unless one met his standards, one's rotation on his service was likely to be a very close approximation of a living hell. Further, even if one met his standards but was on his wrong side—as Carter was to become—then the standards changed in such a way that one could not meet them. It was on the Baker Service, after repeatedly watching Arthur in action, that I developed the concept of quasi-normative error.

Quasi-normative errors are eccentric and attending-specific. Each attending has certain protocols that he[sic] and he[sic] alone follows. A subordinate who does not follow these rules mocks his superordinate's authority; his behavior is a claim that his judgment is as adequate as his superior's; and even though

in no absolute sense can one claim that a mistake has been
made, a subordinate who makes a quasi-normative error risks
his reputation as a trustworthy recruit (61).

Later in the text, in the chapter already discussed with regard to Jones,
"Climbing the Pyramid," I spent a considerable amount of time analyzing the case of Josh Carter. In the promotion meeting in which Jones
was determined to be unfit to continue, Carter was said to be an example of the head-strong type of resident who made quasi-normative errors and, as a result, failed to be retained in the training program. In the
chapter, Carter's problems were seen entirely as a consequence of
Carter's own doings. During the meeting, attendings praised Carter as
an individual of great promise, talent, and ability. At the same time, he
was criticized for being on occasion unreliable, untrustworthy, slovenly, and churlish. When I mentioned to an attending after the meeting
that some of the criticism of Carter seemed to me petty, he responded,
"Just because it's trivial, doesn't mean it is unimportant."

Although I was certainly aware of them for I had witnessed them, I
did not discuss anywhere in the text of *Forgive and Remember* the
provocations under which Carter and his peers worked. By not doing
so I undermined my own intent in developing the concept of quasi-
normative error. My intent, as I understood it at the time, was to show
that the world of surgery was a highly authoritarian one and that that
authority had a defect—it was occasionally eccentric, arbitrary, and
capricious. Yet by not showing the degree to which Carter and others
were baited, I lodge the defect not in authority itself, but in underlings
who are too dim to discern its workings.

Looking back, I think I can see why I might have done so. I wanted
my work to read differently than other sociological accounts of the
time which seemed to engage routinely and somewhat unreflexively in
doctor-bashing. I felt that to present the most extreme examples of
boorish behavior from my field notes would draw attention away from
the book's central thesis—that in surgical education technical norms
are subordinated to moral ones. I worried that parading Arthur's excesses—and Arthur, when I knew him, was a man of excesses—would
draw attention away from the serious side of surgery and, for that matter, of Arthur. In the end, Arthur's colleagues tolerated his excesses be-

cause they recognized that they stemmed from his commitment to excellence and they recognized as well how closely his own performance as a surgeon approached that excellence. At the same time, Arthur's excellence was very much a tightly wound coil; picking at any loose end was a risky and explosive activity. In the end, I behaved like Arthur's colleagues—I forgave him his trespasses. I was appalled and I was charmed. I was only skilled enough as an ethnographic draftsman to present the charmed side.

But there are two problems with this that I now clearly see. First, my behavior, as well as the behavior of Arthur's colleagues, challenges my central thesis about the dominance of normative over technical standards. After all, Arthur's behavior was a normative abomination. We would not tolerate it now. I should not have been silent about it then. To be fair to myself, the text makes the point quite plainly that senior surgeons are not subject to the same rules as residents. It does talk about variation in attending style. But I think that this is all too coy, too clever by half. Second, I feel uneasy about Jones and Carter. The text makes them out to be social incompetents of a sort. They are too simple to figure out the rules of the game. Their problems then are of their own making. Yet this is neither entirely so nor entirely fair. So, I sometimes feel guilty about my treatment of these two residents. There are two dimensions of this guilt worth mentioning here. Most obviously, there is the breaking of generational ranks. I betrayed my peers. In addition, I sided with the aggressor. I know that this is a common enough thing to do in a total institution. All the same I'm not proud.

Some Concluding Remarks, or Why I Told These Stories

Why tell these stories now, so long after they occurred? Why sully Arthur's reputation as a surgeon or my own as a field-worker? Absolution might be one reason that I am choosing now "to put on a hairshirt," but I do not think it is the principal one despite the quite obvious cathartic effect for me of what I have written. I tell these stories now to point out some difficulties embedded in storytelling for didactic purposes. I certainly wanted to emphasize that what stories we choose to tell from our field notes and how we choose to tell them has important consequences. But there is more, I want the re-visioning of the occupational ethics of surgeons presented here to trace some of the fuzzy boundary between the established domain of cultural ethnography and the emerging one of narrative bioethics. I want to suggest why ethnography is not as likely, as some have hoped, to save the life of bioethics (Hoffmaster, 1992).

In writing *Forgive and Remember*, one of my goals was social portraiture. The introduction to *Forgive and Remember* sets two goals for "analytical" ethnography to follow. "First, I want to recapture and refine the old Durkheimian insight that each occupational group possesses its own morality. I want to specify what for the surgeon is the complex of ideas and sentiments, [the] ways of seeing and [of] feeling, [the] certain intellectual and moral framework distinctive of the entire group.... [Second I want to] inform policy by grounding it in a firm understanding of how participants construct their social worlds. It is only from this concrete understanding of the present practical order that any changes in the existing interactional politics of social control can be negotiated" (pp. 5–6). *Forgive and Remember* is medical sociology, an ethnographic description of a professional group's "occupational morals." It is not neutral about those morals; suggestions for improving them are found in the conclusion. On the one hand, in researching and writing *Forgive and Remember*, I strained to provide as detached, neutral, and objective account as possible. Yet, on the other hand, I quite clearly fell short of this goal: with all the talk of "the moral order," "normative codes," and "blameworthy and blameless error," *Forgive and Remember* has a point of view; it can just as easily be read as applied social ethics as empirical social science, as prescriptive and normative as descriptive and empirical.

With these alternative readings in my mind, I presented the two omissions as a device for showing how problematic using ethnographic data for narrative ethics is, for discussing how different the role of bioethicist is from that of ethnographer, and for suggesting some guidelines for writing ethnographies that are "good to think with" either as a social scientist or bioethicist. Before moving on to those tasks, I need to clarify how I assess each of the omissions. The switching of gender, transforming Jones from her to him, strikes me now as a blameworthy error. The error is blameworthy for any number of reasons but most notably, because it makes the text less "good to think with." The very absence of women from the ranks of either attending surgeons or residents should have served as a clue that something worth discussing was out of kilter in the social world whose ethics I was describing. At the same time, I see leaving out the second omission—Arthur's ethnic, religious, and racial slurs—as trivial. I had provided more than enough evidence to suggest that Arthur was difficult to work for, easy to anger, and arbitrary in his judgments. I had also provided more than enough evidence that these faults were not Arthur's alone among senior surgeons, as well as evidence that residents found that the conditions of their employ were stressful. Leaving out the incident in the operating room did not make the ethnography any less good to think with. Including it, however, might have had that effect. It was so startling, so beyond the ordinary, and so offensive that the real danger existed that this behavioral outlier would skew the interpretation of the data. The incident was probably the single most offensive scene I observed during my year and a half of observation. My own sense of propriety, decorum, and fairness suggested to me that I would not want some observing other to hold up for inspection my most offensive professional behavior over the same time period.[7]

If that is so, why tell the second tale now? First, as a simple discursive strategy, the second vignette reinforces the point of the first: if the conditions that the men worked under included such coarse verbal harassment, then imagine what things must have been like for the

7. Beyond all that, the thought occurs that I did not find extreme verbal abuse by authority shocking or extraordinary. It was certainly part of the all-male public high school that I attended. Coaches on any team that I played on indulged in it quite frequently. Faculty at the college that I attended were not shy about dressing students down in class. I think that I expected senior surgeons to be verbally abusive. I was no more shocked by this than I would have been by an abusive army drill instructor. This kind of verbal abuse was not an unusual occurrence in male settings.

The very fact that I did not make much of verbal harassment is yet another reason why I did not make much of Jones' hostile work environment. After all the hostility was not created by gender; it existed for everyone. However, as the lone woman, Jones may have experienced that verbal harassment differently than her male peers who were able to use each other for comfort and support.

women. For this point, I did not have direct evidence. Jones, remember, was a socially isolated woman in a group of men. She trusted me and spoke with me no more than she did with any of the other males around. At that time, I had not honed my own skills well enough to talk with a subject as marginalized and as vulnerable as Jones. Nor had I mastered ethnographic technique well enough to skillfully display reports of what did not happen, what was never observed, what was not asked and answered. So the second omission is told here to make the point of the first omission creditable: that had I paid attention to gender I might have noticed that the operation and application of quasinormative standards undermines the formal fairness of the normative order of surgical training.

There is a second reason to remedy both omissions now. We have known for quite some time that ethnographic narratives are socially constructed, that they are told this way rather than that, that they privilege some voices rather than others. I have also said that the unchallenged voice of authority in the original version of *Forgive and Remember* is the attending surgeon. The epilogue discusses some of the changes that have occurred now that the voice of attending authority is no longer quite so unchallenged. In this commentary, I want to suggest some natural troubles of ethics presented as ethnography or ethnography presented as ethics.

Framing this as a discussion at the boundary between narrative ethics and cultural ethnography imperfectly reframes it as a discussion between cultural insiders and outsiders. By and large those that practice any brand of narrative ethics base their claims to expertise, their special purchase on affairs, to some sort of "insider" status. By the same token, those who produce ethnographies of medicine base their claims to expertise, their special purchase on affairs, on their "outsider" status: lacking any stake in immediate outcomes permits continued neutrality, makes objective observation and analysis possible.

When I began the research for *Forgive and Remember*, I was an outsider at Pacific Hospital. Not only that, I was fairly certain that by the time the research was published, I would no longer be at Pacific. I would only have a few sentimental ties to Pacific Hospital's Department of Surgery. At the beginning of the research, I was an outsider who knew nothing of hospitals or of residency training. As the research went on, I learned things; and, as I learned things, I became more of an "insider," but there was always a "responsibility barrier"—I never had to make decisions and do things on behalf of others. As the research progressed, I developed relationships, made friends, and built up obligations. These all affected what stories I chose to tell and how I chose to tell them. In my own eyes, I was there to reveal how some of the backstage of surgery was connected to its public presentation. That became the general narrative guideline (save for Jones's gender) for constructing *Forgive and Remember*. On rereading the text, I am struck at what I chose to leave out the first time around, and the cool detached tone through which events are narrated, judgments made, and solutions proposed.

Narrative ethics is generally practiced by insiders in health care. Some are employed in hospitals in other clinical roles, some are hired purely for their expertise as ethicists to sit on hospital committees, provide in-service, continuing and public education, contribute to research, and consult on difficult cases. In this work they develop relationships, make friends, juggle multiple responsibilities, and build up obligations. All of this work is done in an organizational environment in which strong professional norms of confidentiality exist and are routinely breached. If narrative ethicists wish to produce public ethnographic accounts of their work, they will need to trade on those relationships, betray some of those friendships, ignore some of their ethical obligations, and tread, however lightly, on those norms of confidentiality. The very work of telling stories, which may very well involve the public airing of some dirty organizational linen, may then transform insiders into outsiders in health care settings. Those with tales to tell may find themselves as frozen out of the everyday discourse as Jones was. This, then, may compromise their effectiveness as clinical workers in other domains, ethics committee members, or consultants.

All of this is to say that the intersection of ethnography, narrative, and ethics is vexed. The space between objective description and involved activity is closer than we might think if we are looking in the rearview mirror alone. Ethnographers can not retreat from studies of contested ethical situations. Our credentials as outsiders or insiders need to be continually negotiated and renegotiated. We need to think more complexly than we have about where the line that separates observer effect and the legitimate exercise of expertise is, how we will know we have crossed it, and how we will know when such crossings are not just permissible but compulsory. Narrative ethicists also have to think about the tradeoffs in their work as well, about when to argue and when to let go, and when to make a public issue of a private trouble.[8] For both ethnographers and narrative ethicists, how much of the backstage to reveal is a recurring question. How each answers that question is a function of how each defines the professional, the public, and the collective dimension of their role responsibilities. For cultural ethnographers as for narrative ethicists, social obligations and a sense of skill at meeting them spring from self-definition and from the paired questions: Why am I here and what am I doing?

The body of this appendix is a telling of stories I chose not to tell once upon a time. I pulled my punches even though I had no institutional interests to safeguard, no individuals that I needed to protect, and no agenda that I sought to promote. Even with that, as a moral tale, an example of applied ethics, *Forgive and Remember* is a thickly described, thin story. The thick description is in the everyday account of the resident's life and professional vulnerabilities. The thin story is the account that does not more strongly question all the prerogatives claimed in the name of attending authority. This defect also suggests a remedy for those that engage in some form of applied ethics, whether ethnographic or narrative, theoretic or applied. We need to ask ourselves: how many voices we have allowed to speak and how many hidden presumptions we have questioned. One mode of doing this for both ethnographers and narrative ethicists is to revisit our work from time to time and ask How would we act differently now, what story would we tell this time?

8. This is Mills' formula and it remains a good one to think with. As everyday actors, those who practice clinical ethics need a keen sense of the sociological imagination. One way to assure such an imagination is collaborative projects that are multi-sited.

Works Cited

Bosk, Charles L. 1992. *All God's Mistakes: Genetic Counseling in a Pediatric Hospital*. Chicago: University of Chicago Press.

Bosk, Charles L. 2001. "Irony, Ethnography, and In Informed Consent." In *Bioethics in Social Context*, edited by Barry C. Hoffmaster. Philadelphia: Temple University Press, pp. 199–220.

Chambers, Tod. 1999. *The Fiction of Bioethics: Cases as Literary Texts*. New York: Routledge.

Davis, Dena. 1991. "Rich Cases: The Ethics of Thick Description." *Hastings Center Report* 21: 12–17.

Epilogue

Recently, I received two invitations to give public lectures. The first came from a group of ethicists and medical educators who had read *Forgive and Remember* when it first appeared. They thought a statement of how the argument of the book now needed to be modified in light of all the changes in American society and culture over the last twenty years, most particularly those that have impacted on health care, would make for an interesting discussion. The second invitation came from a young assistant professor of surgery at a state medical school in the heartland, who had just read *Forgive and Remember*. He thought the book captured his residency perfectly. He could not believe that someone writing about another program in another place at another time described so well the ordeal that he had just completed. Fresh from a visit to his chair, he had a simple request: Would I be a visiting professor of surgery sometime in the fall? He asked that I spend a few days lecturing on *Forgive and Remember*—its lessons were so timely, so unchanging that this would be a service to residents. Later, when I spoke with his chair, he too said a visit would be beneficial. He had just had to let go a number of residents, morale was low, trust had deteriorated—he said it would be a good time to refresh everybody on the "rules of the game."

So, in the space of a few days, I was asked to update an argument that time had frayed, and I was asked to repeat that same argument because of its timeless aspects. The burden of this epilogue is to demonstrate how both assessments are valid. The general insights of *Forgive and Remember* are in need of revision and yet timeless. The world of residents is very much as I described it—there is still the same time-pressured ordeal of learning by doing, there is still the same personal vulnerability that comes from a never-ending series of competence tests that then determine the trajectory of a professional career, there is still the same dangerous social placement betwixt and between professional infancy and professional adulthood. These are constants and no amount of social reorganization will change these aspects of the resident's status. At the same time, the world of the attending has changed. The attending of *Forgive and Remember*, an absolute and not always benign despot, who needs merely to speak to command resources and action, is largely a figure of the past. While we might have predicted that this diminution of the attending's authority would have improved the resident's position, it did not—in the world of surgery, power and authority are no longer the simple two-person, zero-sum game that *Forgive and Remember* describes. If anything, the diminution of attending authority has worsened the resident's position.

The hydraulics of excrement, or the social plumbing of "organizational troubles," explain how as the absolute despotism of attendings decreased, the vulnerabilities of residents increased. When I was researching *Forgive and Remember*, I heard more times than I ever recorded in my field notes—and I recorded it there quite a lot—the not-so-scholarly adage, "shit rolls downstream." As the attending finds his/her authority challenged by many competing social forces, the difficulties of resolving these often conflicting social expectations get passed on to residents. The nature of these demands, the new order of the hospital, is the theme of this epilogue.

More Than Twenty Years Ago Today

Before describing how the world has changed, I need to briefly describe the world of surgery and academic medicine as I found it. In rereading *Forgive and Remember*, I discovered a humbling social principle: when social scientists can describe clearly a social world, when we can sketch precisely the lineaments of a social structure, then that structure is bound to change and to change relatively quickly. Were this not so, the features of the social structure would not be so well defined, so easy to isolate. Perhaps it is the case that structure becomes visible when systems are under stress and when cycles of reform have begun.[1]

---

1. While there was little agitation for reform in residency at Pacific during my fieldwork other places were beginning to see the formation of house staff unions. More sig-

When formerly unquestioned assumptions become targets of reform, both their challengers and defenders create and learn a vocabulary to describe both things as they are and things as they could become. This process of verbalization makes the sociologist's job easier, making structures and dynamics easier to see; but it also suggests that when the stress points become visible, the system is disintegrating. The illusion of a stable system is a bit like the motionlessness of a roller coaster at the apex of its ascent before the plunge. *Forgive and Remember* does a creditable job describing a type of power and authority at its apex; however, it does a very poor job of predicting the next moment, the plunge.

The lost world of power and authority that *Forgive and Remember* describes so well is one in which an unlimited *clinical individualism* reigns with virtually no checks or limits. Ostensibly, the text is about the socialization of young residents around the issue of mistakes, a narrative about how a professional conscience is forged in the crucible of training. As the book unfolds we see how young residents learn what is a blameless and what is a blameworthy error. We see, in addition, the teaching faculty of attending surgeons model a professional conscience by "putting on a hair shirt" and confessing mistakes to an assembled collegium in the weekly Mortality and Morbidity Conference. The book moves from morning rounds to operating room, to conference room, to cafeteria to show how lessons about mistakes and errors, professional obligations and responsibilities, as well as personal sacrifice and limits are embedded in everyday routines. All of these routines involve a dictatorial, authoritarian attending and a near-powerless resident, chafing at the unfairness of it all.

---

nificant, critical first-person accounts of postgraduate medical training were being published as mass market books for the first time.

Beyond that, critiques of overly expensive, overly technological care were being voiced. There was also a nascent movement, expressed through newly mandated Peer Standards Review Organizations (PSRO) to make physicians more accountable for the quality of care they render.

So at the time of the fieldwork, sentiments of reform were in the air, so to speak. They had not yet landed on the ground in a way that affected the everyday activities of surgeons.

More than twenty tears later, however compelling this description of a once-hidden social world remains, it has one glaring defect—the description appears both too simple and too isolated from the larger world of which it was but a part. This intense focus gives the text a certain power but is in itself an odd defect in a piece of sociology. For sociologists, the academic medical center has long been the paradigm of the complex, bureaucratically administered, formal organization. Yet the world of *Forgive and Remember* is so very different. It is a hermetically sealed environment of a work group comprised of imperious attendings and cowering residents, with patients as nothing more than just so much raw material. There is no mention of meddlesome administrators, arbitrary insurers, or avaricious attorneys. The omnipresent concern for what "third parties" might think—something I observed studying genetic counselors not even a full ten years later—was nowhere to be found. If a third party was mentioned in surgery, it was only to dismiss the relevance of whatever they might offer. In the world of *Forgive and Remember*, health care is not managed, it is dictated. Those who are doing that dictating are the attending surgeons of Pacific Hospital.

The power and authority of these attendings is the major leitmotif of *Forgive and Remember*. The attending who occupies the most central role in the text is Dr. Arthur. It was never clear if Dr. Arthur came to surgery from his residency or from central casting. A commanding presence, Dr. Arthur was ramrod straight, immaculately groomed whether in starched greens or streetclothes, and insufferably self-assured—so definite were all of his pronouncements that his residents usually remarked, without irony, that it was if everything he said came directly from God. Dr. Arthur had both a sense of humor and a touch of cruelty; and when these were combined with a resident as the target, the life of that resident became the operational definition of misery. Finally, as an example of one of those confusions that make it hard to say whether life imitates art or the reverse, Dr. Arthur (who had been a battlefield surgeon in Korea) dispayed the same attitude to formal bureaucratic authority and acted out the same mixture of contempt and subversion that characterized the surgeons on the TV series *M.A.S.H.*, which was a top-rated show when I was in the field gathering my data.

The other attending who occupies a central role in the text is Dr.

White, whom I used as a foil to Dr. Arthur. White was as relaxed as Arthur was intense, as self-effacing as Arthur was self-promoting, as gentle as Arthur was harsh, as rumpled as Arthur was sartorially splendid. If Dr. Arthur appeared every inch the archetypal surgeon, then Dr. White was cast against type. A quiet and reflective man, Dr. White and I often conversed at the conclusion of a day's procedures in the fading twilight of the surgeons' lounge about the limits, problems, and shortcomings of American medicine as practiced in elite academic centers at the beginning of the last quarter of the twentieth century. Dr. White fretted about many things: the rising costs of services, the multiple problems of providing care for the indigent, the future of the service ideal, the ethics of cutting-edge surgery, and the declining public trust in professional authority. Such conversations were impossible to imagine with Arthur, who never appeared to acknowledge doubt about anything save for the sanity of those with the temerity to disagree with him.

But the contrast between Dr. Arthur and Dr. White really served to demonstrate a distinction without a difference. For what Arthur and White shared was much more important than what separated them. These surgeons shared, along with all their colleagues at Pacific Hospital, an unshakeable commitment to the omnipotent authority of the attending surgeon in matters of organizing his (at the time there were no women attendings) service. The range of claims made in the name of an individual's clinical autonomy was quite broad. It included: the ability to overrule courses of treatment indicated by the scientific literature based on clinical authority; the right to decide what to do in ethically problematic situations; and the judgment of whether a resident's shortcomings were excusable or not.

To give a sense of how extensive this clinical individualism and authority once were and to foreshadow the remainder of this discussion, let me quote extensively from a field excerpt presented in *Forgive and Remember*. I am fond of telling my students that data never speaks for itself, but here may be the exception that proves the rule. As I present this case, think for yourself how differently it would be managed today. Think also of how many of the unquestioned assumptions of decision making in the elite medical center have changed since the mid-1970s. In *Forgive and Remember*, there is no commentary on any of the ethi-

cal dimensions of the case, save for the spare observation that there is
no discussion after the attending's soliloquy and that this absence of
discussion leaves the attending's decision and his reasons for it unexplored. I use this terse observation of the attending's long publically
spoken justification for his decision making as evidence to support the
assertion that the norm of heroic intervention is so deeply embedded in
surgery that its breach requires explanation. I found nothing in the assertion of authority, the process of decision making, worthy of special
commentary. The scene is the weekly Mortality and Morbidity Conference. What follows is a reconstructed but nearly verbatim account by
one senior surgeon of one child's death:

> Dr. Porter, a pediatric surgeon, stepped forward to present the
> third case himself, mumbling as he walked to the front of the
> room, "I think I'd better take care of this myself." He began:
> "This third case is very different from the first two presented.
> Where the first two cases involve questions of patient selection
> and the taking of risk to prolong life, cases where everything
> must go right if the surgical intervention is to succeed, this third
> case involves the taking of risk not to prolong life. This is a de-
> cision that only an attending physician can make and for which
> he alone is responsible. This infant was born with "prune belly"
> [wrinkling of skin on the belly from absence of abdominal mus-
> cles], complete atresia of the urethra [closing of outflow from
> urinary bladder], various deformities of the legs and feet which
> may have been the result of the fetus's position and may have
> been corrected with time, an omphalocele [a large hernia at the
> umbilicus] and a heart murmur. The obstetrician and the pedia-
> trician at the hospital where the infant was born put the baby
> aside to die; but, as luck would have it, it did not. They then
> called me up to arrange a transfer. They both expressed the
> hope that the baby would die, but in my hands. Here is where
> the situation gets complicated. The mother is a thirty-year-old
> woman. She married at twenty-six and put off conception a
> number of years while she was under psychiatric care. Then she
> had some trouble conceiving and finally she had this baby. She
> had never seen the child. The father, acting with the obstetrician
> and the pediatrician, had arranged the transfer and supported
> the decision not to make heroic efforts to save the child's life.

I thought we had to be straightforward enough in this case to inform the mother of the baby's problems because of the psychological aspects of the mother-child, mother-father, doctor-patient relationship, as well as our various legal responsibilities. So I did the minimum necessary to give the baby a chance until the mother could see it. I repaired the omphalecele. The mother did come up and see the baby. She was obviously under heavy sedation and quite difficult to deal with. She waxed and waned in her support of the child. She couldn't decide if the baby should survive. It was then that I decided that the baby should not be considered for cardiac arrest treatment, and that no urgent or emergency measures should be taken to save the baby's life. These children need total support if they are to have any chance at all. This baby would never be normal and without the total support of both parents there was no hope for a satisfactory adjustment. I have seen many marriages totally disrupted by the extensive hospitalization that such cases require after a number of years. This is why I decided to let the infant die. This is, as I said before, a decision that only an attending can make. It is needless to say a very difficult decision. Yet in this case it is one that I'm totally comfortable with" (132–34).

To state that much has changed is to belabor the obvious—to state that the process today would be far different, that it would involve hospital attorneys and ethics committees, that there would be a more elaborated discussion, and a more carefully thought-out rationale upon which a decision would be bottomed is to simply describe what that change has been. In the remainder of this epilogue, I wish to describe both those changes and the social forces behind them.

Clinical Individualism
Redux

One of the first jokes I heard about surgeons had as its punchline— "That's God, he thinks he's a surgeon." This joke was but one of many I heard during my fieldwork to poke fun at surgeons' vanity, pride, and sense of self-importance. In *Forgive and Remember*, I am quite tolerant of surgeons' egos and their vanities. I point out that they may be necessary if surgeons are to engage in the kind of hubristic action that is major surgery. While surgeons' personalities may not have changed so much over the last twenty years, surgeons are themselves much less likely to be the topic of medical humor. My admittedly subjective impression is that the focus of humor is now predominantly administrators of managed care plans. This shift is itself one indication of the decline in importance of clinical individualism and the concomitant increase of bureaucratic management at the bedside.

Managed Care and the Surgeon

So many others have spent so much time explaining the coming of managed care and corporate values to American medicine that there is little to be gained here by rehearsing those discussions. All that needs to be emphasized is that two general presuppositions of any regime of managed care clash with the ethos of surgery as I found it in the 1970s, namely (1) that resources should be utilized more efficiently and (2) that this efficiency can be obtained through centralized decision making far from the bedside.

First, surgery was not organized in the mid-70s to model the efficient use of resources. Rather, surgery exemplified the extravagant mobilization of resources for individual salvage. This was the heroic ideal. Quite explicitly, the norm that covered action was—do everything possible, whatever is necessary to prolong life is required, save for very special circumstances. We have already seen, in the case of the damaged neonate presented above, that any breaches of this rule were seen to be so extraordinary as to require special explanation. The rule—do everything, never mind the cost—was communicated in a number of different ways. It was explicitly stated whenever residents were dressed down for performance that failed to meet expectations. The benefits of adherence to the rule were commented upon each time some patient who had survived long odds returned to the outpatient clinic and was displayed to the workgroup as a living example of what utmost dedication means. Arthur communicated the rules through the extravagant hours that he worked—each time he left the operating room after a twelve- or fourteen-hour day, he would pull off his gloves and address the rest of the team still closing the patient's surgical wound, "Well, gentlemen, we certainly earned our pay today." The rest of the team was aware that however true the statement, it was only Arthur's day that was ending. For the rest of the team, the day was far from over: the surgery was not complete, there was still a wound to close and post-op orders to write, there was still the wait in the recovery room area, and there were still rounds to be made on the rest of the services' patients. Arthur, of course, knew that; and both he and the residents knew that his and their salary were unaffected by the number of hours that they worked.

In many ways, much of the satisfaction of surgery at Pacific derived from individual physicians, going beyond what was expected to achieve unexpected success. Self-sacrifice, a distaste for any calculation of cost and benefit, a willingness to run long odds on the patient's behalf—all of these characterized the surgical personality. The ethos was anti-bureaucratic, anti-rules, and, if need be, anti-rational, especially if rationality were measured in terms of cost-benefit ratios, expectancies, and likely outcomes. Any limitation of effort, any expressions of doubt, any hesitation before action, any anxiety about success—all these were seen as alien to the true surgeon. Around the time of *Forgive and Remember*'s publication, Tom Wolfe's book *The Right Stuff* appeared. I was struck, as were a number of reviewers of *Forgive and Remember*, by how similar the culture of test pilots and academic surgeons appeared to be. The consequences of timidity, of hesitation, of staying too securely within the edge of the envelope were to lose the respect of peers, to fail to be recognized as a "true surgeon."

Lest the reader think that I romanticize this ethos too much, let me state that I was fully aware of its downside: the futile attempts to save life that only multiplied suffering; the absence of anything like genuine informed consent as patients' doubts were overwhelmed by attendings' optimism; the abusive environment created whenever residents' or nurses' efforts failed to be as extravagantly heroic as their superiors would have wished; and the personal costs to individuals of prolonged subjection to these abusive conditions. In general, I was aware enough of the almost tragic conditions created by the socially structured and socially reinforced inability to accept limits that I compared surgeons' reactions to death, especially unexpected death, to that of prideful Achilles repairing to his tent. In my files somewhere, I have a paper that I have been too timid to publish titled, "Residency as Training for Impairment," that discusses how the lessons learned in residency may exact unintended negative consequences as they extend through the life course. To describe a heroic ideal is not to endorse it.

But, awareness of that downside notwithstanding, there was something sociologically (and even personally) appealing in the surgeons' modeling of the fiduciary relationship in its idealized and even in its grotesque forms. That appeal is nothing more complex than the clarity with which it revealed the indispensable, irrationally excessive element of professional service. Seeing this so clearly reminds us of the real challenge of managed care—harmonizing the values of the service ideal with those of economic efficiency. And we can specify this challenge further for academic surgery. If we assume that the surgical personality exists for a reason, that it serves some need connected to treating bodies in this aggressive way to heal them, then how does that personality coexist with a management regime hostile to its assumptions, its expression, and even its definition of success? How does the physician's fiduciary responsibility to the individual patient get dramatized in a management regime committed to the most efficient collective deployment of resources? How do young apprentices learn about necessary personal sacrifice for another at the same time that they learn to be efficient resource managers?

Whether it is through shorter lengths of stay, more rigidly prescribed indications for surgery, more tightly controlled pharmaceutical formularies, or more careful surveillance of surgeons' practice profiles—each and every one of the management practices associated with managed care undercut the authority and unchallenged clinical individualism of the attending surgeon. As we shall see in a moment, this diminution in the authority of the attending does little to improve the lot of the resident. In fact, it contributes to the resident's greater immiseration. Before describing how this happens, we need to look at one additional change in the hospital environment since I wrote *Forgive and Remember*, a change that further undermines the power and authority of the attending surgeon.

The New Moral Authority at the Bedside

When I started my research for *Forgive and Remember*, like most members of American society, I had never heard of bioethicists. And when, toward the end of research, I became aware of the word and the role associated with it, I was highly skeptical of any success for the enterprise, especially in the world of surgery. Surgeons were so impatient around problems that lacked clear solutions, so impatient of talk, so eager for action. Bioethics seemed so abstract and value-laden while the clinical dilemmas of medicine seemed so concrete and so demanding of action in such an immediate present. I did not see how the style of bioethicists would ever mesh with the style of clinical medicine.

My skepticism about bioethics was coupled with an awareness of the moral or ethical problems associated with academic medicine. *Forgive and Remember* discusses among other issues the difficulties surgeons have recognizing the end of life; the problems they have managing it humanely once they recognize it; the obstacles to a genuinely voluntary informed consent; and the various, yet quotidian, assaults on the dignity of the patient as a person. *Forgive and Remember* did pay attention to what we would now call the bioethics of surgery—how could I study mistakes and not do so? The attention was relentlessly empirical—here is the problem, this is what the various parties did, and these are the reasons they gave to explain their behavior. Nowhere do I make the move from the empirical to the normative: this is what the parties should do, here are the principles they should apply, and these are the values that should be privileged. As a sociologist, I had been trained to pay attention to what is and not to make judgments about what should be.

The normative features of the empirical world that I was attempting to describe were not very structurally complex. The patient was etherized upon a table. The attending surgeon was the sole decision maker. There was no formal requirement at the time to have any particular decision inspected, debated, justified, or evaluated. But Pacific Hospital was an academic institution; and this created, at best, a subtle pressure for collective reflection. After all, the quality of teaching and the seriousness of professional education depended on how much attendings were willing to define certain situations as problematic, clinically or morally; how much they were willing to share of their reasoning or "philosophy"; and how open they were to entertaining approaches alternative to their own.

There was instruction for the residents around the ethics of clinical care. Such instruction took place only on those occasions when attendings determined it was necessary, and only then, when the press of other work did not interfere. Pedagogically the system was not without its flaws. First, the resources for anyone who wished to question attending action were quite limited. Residents possessed, as their only weapon, the gentle question; both nurses and patients appeared to lack even this. Next, questions were entertained at the discretion of the attending, who therefore also had the power to ignore them as well as the ability to express displeasure at those who raised pointless questions that wasted time. Residents or students who were seen as excessively preoccupied with moral matters were seen as not possessing a "surgical personality"; the fear of being so labeled was a major deterrent to any open conversation. In general, ethical questions were seen as sinkholes for time which could otherwise be spent productively; the distaste for discussion of ethical questions was bottomed on the fact that there was no "gold standard" for resolving these question, no clear guideposts for preferring one approach to another. The general take on ethics was that each resident needed to develop his or her philosophy so that once he or she became an attending, he or she could translate that philosophy into action. Philosophies, approaches, or styles could be developed from observations of attending behavior and the spare rationales that occasionally accompanied that action. Never was there any suggestion that the ethical dilemmas of surgery required anything more for their resolution than the decisive intervention of the attending surgeon.

So the ethics of treatment is a second area where the clinical individualism of the attending has been eroded. The reasons for this are many—the extensions of the civil-rights movement to patients as a category of disenfranchised person, the decline in the moral authority of the medical profession as a result of well-publicized abuses in research and in the clinic, and the disconnect between what Eliot Mischler has called the "lifeworld" of the patient and the "lifeworld" of medicine. However the rise of bioethics is explained, all of the structures that have been put into place as a consequence undercut the previously unchallenged authority of the attending surgeon. We now have a more muscular concept of informed consent and patient autonomy, the Patient Self-Determination Act, the Do Not Resuscitate Order, the living will, the durable power of attorney, and the clinical ethics consultation service and the institutional ethics committee. None of these existed when I did the research for *Forgive and Remember*. Back then, a requirement such as that of the Joint Commission on the Accreditation of Health Care Organizations, stating that all health care organizations have in place a mechanism for the resolution of ethical conflict was unthinkable because unnecessary—the judgment of attending physicians was sufficient for the resolution of any and all conflicts.

Now, despite all this structural change, we probably should not rush to the judgment that merely because the intent of all this activity has been to level the playing field that this is, in fact, what has occurred. It is certainly undeniable that nurses have greater resources for challenging physicians by relabeling as "ethical" those disagreements involving power and authority in the workplace. It is not debatable that there are a new variety of procedural requirements to assure ethical action. However, we lack evidence to document the impact of all this activity. In fact, we do not even know what to count as evidence about the impact of all these changes because we are so unclear about their goals. For example, has the goal of all this structural change been to secure patient rights, insulate hospitals from liability, or insure that the proper decision is made?

Beyond that, most of the structural change that has occurred is premised on a model that assumes decision making among equally rational actors. However, with the distinct exception of some chronically-ill patients, feeling lost, disoriented, confused, and frightened is an irreducible part of the experience of illness. Any rationalizing model for medical decision making that does not take into account the fact that many patients and their families cannot negotiate effectively precisely because they are sick and because the family is overwhelmed by the existential reality of life-threatening illness is bound to fail at leveling the playing field. In addition, merely because problems can be described as ethical does not mean that this will be the case. During my fieldwork, patients that were resistant to the treatment plans of physicians or who frustrated their caretakers were often classified as having psychiatric problems rather than as having made different value choices than their surgeons. On surgery services, psychiatric or psychological diagnoses were not seen as hypotheses worthy of investigation and treatment in their own right. Rather, these diagnoses were used to stigmatize patients and to dismiss their objections. Having structures in place to contest decisions on ethical grounds does not mean that those structures will be utilized. Still, there are procedures, structures, and personnel that exist for challenging attending authority that did not exist when I did my fieldwork.

Residency Redux

With the authority of the attending surgeon challenged both as to its clinical and moral base, we might think the capacity of attendings to tyrannize residents, to control their lives, to shape their behaviors, and to control their futures has been reduced. This has not happened. In fact, I think the opposite has occurred, that the world of the resident is a much less happy, more highly stressed one than it was twenty years ago, and it was not all that happy or unstressed then. Oddly enough it is the deflation of the attending's power and authority that has made the resident's lot worse. So here we have a peculiar paradox to explain: if the attending's unlimited power was the source of such misery for residents, how is it that a reduction in that authority created even more misery?

The answer lies partly in what these changes have meant for the day-to-day operation of a surgical service and partly in how residents are evaluated by attending surgeons. Many of the changes of managed care have in essence been the operational equivalent of speeding up the assembly line. If hospital stays are shorter and if service size is constant, then those patients being treated are sicker as a group than they were twenty years ago. We speak of this glibly when we speak of how the acuity index is now higher than it once was. What we do not stop to consider is what this means for the day-to-day responsibilities of residents. Sicker patients require more surveillance, more management, more worry, more coordination with nursing, more consulting with colleagues in other specialties, more scheduling of ancillary services, and more communication with family members than do less sick ones. To these stresses we can add one set of others—managed care requires more negotiations, more preauthorizations, more formal bureaucratic requirements than the previous laissez-faire regime of "doctor knows best." A good many of these requirements fall upon residents' shoulders. And even when they do not, the failure to comply with them does. In the residency that I observed, no one was ever surprised when blame, like excrement, ran downstream.

The erosion of the moral authority of the attending has had the same consequences as the erosion of clinical authority. Now the appropriateness of action is open to multiple challenges. Think of all the different ways a surgeon's course of action can be challenged and all the parties that feel both entitled and empowered to make such a challenge. Now think of how few of these routes existed twenty years ago and even if they had, how many fewer parties would have felt entitled to use them. Think how we would receive the assertion today that, "This is a moral decision that an attending surgeon and an attending surgeon alone can make."

The rub of this for residents is that one of the criteria that attendings use to measure a resident's worth is how well they organize and run the service. Operationally what this means is that when the attending is spared the aggravation of disgruntled patients, mutinous nurses, unhappy family members, and apoplectic administrators, he/she then often infers that the resident is doing a good job. A good job means that work runs smoothly and the attending is able to concentrate on the pure work of surgery and surgical research, free from the polluting social concerns and troubles that sometimes arise in the wake of life-threatening illness. If attendings generally infer from a smoothly running service that a resident is competent, they always infer from a poorly running one that a resident is not competent.

Now, running a service smoothly was difficult enough work in the bygone days that *Forgive and Remember* describes. Coordinating tests, retrieving lab results, finding X-rays, managing the post-op period, charting the day's events, keeping medications current, arranging for transport, balancing intake and output, communicating with nurses, scheduling consultations—these labors appeared Herculean at a time when they could be done on healthier patients without intrusion from either clinical, economic, or moral watchdogs. Today, residents are much more vulnerable on a much wider number of fronts. There are just so many more places where leaks can spring in the tight ship they are in charge of running. There are so many more opportunities to be found wanting.

The Unbearable Sameness of Change

I began this epilogue by claiming that part of the argument of *Forgive and Remember* was frayed and part of it was timeless. We can now see clearly exactly how that is so. The conditions under which residents labor and are judged have changed. All of these changes have reduced the power and authority of attending surgeons. Strangely, because attendings are less powerful, the day-to-day challenges that residents must meet have multiplied. Yet, despite having their once near-total authority eroded, attendings are still in a position to be despotic with residents. And, if I were the type to engage in cheap armchair psychologizing, I might argue that their inability to be despotic in other spheres of the hospital might even increase attendings' need to be despotic with residents.

Unchanged in all this, so far as I can tell, are the actual rules by which residents are found wanting. Here the argument of *Forgive and Remember* retains its force. Certain errors are considered blameless—these errors do not stain a recruit's reputation. They merely signal the need for further training. The forgiveness of these errors by attendings creates obligations in residents—the obligation to work harder, to dedicate oneself to patient care, and to improve performance. Other errors are thought of as blameworthy—these errors blemish both the recruit's and, potentially, the profession's reputation. To be found wanting for committing these errors generally signals that the individual had engaged in conduct unbecoming a surgeon. Such errors are evidence that no amount of training can help the individual who makes them. These errors are not forgiven, and those that make them are often extruded from either the training program or surgery. The failure to forgive establishes the normative boundaries for professional behavior. In the last twenty years, this structure for categorizing, judging, and sanctioning errors has not changed, calls to change the culture of "naming, blaming, and shaming" notwithstanding. In fact, the system has grown harsher.

But, there is also the possibility that the apparent stability is masking some very deep fault lines in the moral geology of training. The system for managing error had worked as well as it had for a number of reasons: there had been an unchallenged, unquestioned authority making judgments, there had been a broad social consensus underpinning the authority of those decision makers, and there had been a single interpretation of the service ethic, the duties of a fiduciary. Today none of these conditions continues to apply. The single decision maker has been undercut by the algorithms of managed care and the applied princplism of bioethics; the broad consensus that allowed for the arbitrary exercise of authority has been replaced by a concern for "due process"—and the increasing diversity in the demographics of surgical residency has only heightened this concern; and finally, the single interpretation of the service ethic—do everything possible—has broken down. It is challenged not only by administrators but also by patients and their families who fear that everything may compromise their dignity and multiply their suffering. Under these conditions, the clarity of old norms has broken down and not yet been replaced by a set of norms shared by all.

Notes

Chapter Two

1. The sociological literature on accounts and motives deals with breached expectations. Worthy of special note are Dewey (1922); Lyman and Scott (1968); Foote (1951); Blum and McHugh (1971); and Mills (1944).

2. An acceptable answer in everyday terms is one which renders further questions unnecessary. It ends the search procedure. (See Churchill 1971.)

3. Orderly surgical activity occurs when attending surgeons have their plans carried out with little disruption by deaths and complications—physiological accident—or by others in the work group—social accident.

4. Citations with a name indicate interview material. Citations with service indicate participant-observer data.

5. I am grateful to Edward Shils (1975) for the conceptual imagery. Recently Barber et al. (1973) have questioned Merton's (1957) conception of medical schools as moral leaders. Right or wrong, Barber and his colleagues are somewhat beside the point. Medical schools, as they suggest, may not provide much in the way of moral leadership, but they are the only leadership the next generation of physicians has.

6. See chapter 7.

7. Two good early discussions of uncertainty are Fox (1957) and Davis (1960). Fox discusses how physicians learn to manage uncertainty as students; Davis deals with its control implications in the doctor-patient relationship.

Chapter Three

1. The traffic of rounds provides interesting grist for two of Goffman's mills: vehicular traffic (1971) and deference patterns (1967).

2. Freidson (1970a) discusses these in a different context.

3. Here it is perhaps necessary to remind the reader that a distinctive feature of surgical training is that until one reaches attending status the

direct orders of superordinates are seen as legitimate (see Goss 1961; Stelling and Bucher 1972; and Miller 1970).

4. There is a rich underground lore among surgeons about researchers whose procedures were less than scientific.

5. The distinction between board-certified and occasional surgeons becomes meaningful given the great amount of surgery done by noncertified surgeons in this country. The board-certified surgeons claim that this is a major flaw in our delivery system: they cannot control surgery unless they can control who may act as surgeons. The power to decide who may do surgery is currently in the hands of hospital trustees who are often members of religious or fraternal orders; rarely are they professionals. A few times when I asked Arthur about controls at hospitals other than Pacific, he answered: "Five pounds of candy to Mother Superior at Christmastime will cover a multitude of sins." By which I suppose he meant to make perfectly clear the nonprofessional manner in which work in a hospital is regulated.

Chapter Four

1. Field researchers (see Dalton 1959) have noted this phenomenon— the loose-mouthedness of the malcontent—as a general problem in coding the reliability of information that their field subjects pass on to them. Undoubtedly members of an organization are as aware as field researchers of this, but how they weight information against its source in building up their own interpretation of what is "really" going on is a largely unexplored topic.

2. As subordinates who must account for failure to superordinates are well aware, one person's backstage is another's center. Backstage refers to spaces where actors may retreat and allow some distance between themselves and their roles. I would speculate that the relationship between backstage privacy and status is U-shaped. The very poor, those who command no social resources, cannot afford a backstage area; and the very celebrated are often followed far backstage: Bob Dylan and Henry Kissinger's garbage is ransacked. Jacqueline Onassis and Photographer Ray Gaella bickered in court for quite some time over when public curiosity invades private backstage and becomes a public nuisance. Recently, how far televised news may invade the private spaces of private individuals during public disasters has become a question of journalistic ethics (see *New York Times*, 6 July 1975, Arts and Leisure Section, p. 1).

3. The background resources that participants employ for under-standing such action literally without thinking is the basic problem that ethnomethodology explores. Garfinkel (1967) and his followers (Sudnow [1972] is an especially useful collection) have demonstrated how much work sustains the most ordinary interactions. Such work demonstrates how problematic cell 1 can be when subject to scrutiny. However, I have noticed that the field-workers who take Garfinkel's ideas seriously pay little heed to his chief methodological injunction: "Procedurally, it is my preference to start with familiar scenes and ask what can be done to produce trouble. The operations that one would have to perform in order to multiply the senseless features of the perceived environments to pro-duce and sustain bewilderment, consternation, and confusion; to pro-duce the socially structured effects of anxiety, shame and guilt, and indignation; and to produce disorganized interaction should say some-thing about how the structures of everyday activity are ordinarily produced and maintained" (pp. 37–38). Field-researchers of an ethno-methodological frame of mind do not go out and create troubles— this is reserved for experimentalists (see McHugh 1968)—rather, they ask what participants in a scene see as their normal troubles and how they manage them to create artful interactions (for good examples, see Bittner 1967; Sudnow 1965, 1967; and Emerson 1970). There is in this approach a convergence with Hughes' suggestions for studying occupa-tions and the world of work.

4. Two features of the medical environment are important in under-standing why such questioning occurs as it does. First, there is the depth of the student's unfamiliarity with surgery. The students I observed almost uniformly expressed their surprise at the following: that immed-iately following surgery, previously healthy-looking individuals appeared so sick. Attendings work on convincing them that this is "normal" and "no cause for alarm." Here a few good results go a long way in refocus-ing student concern from patient-oriented to procedure-oriented con-cerns, that is, from worrying about an individual bleeding to the methods used to control bleeding. Second, there is the surgeon's sensi-tivity to the stereotype other specialists hold of him as a mere "tinkerer," a "technician," or a "body plumber." Attendings and residents are well aware of and resent these views. As a result, surgeons spend a great deal of their time demonstrating to students the sophistication of their clinical reasoning. Undoubtedly some of this is encouraged by the academic climate; however, some of it appears as defensive reaction to a negative stereotype.

5. Two digressions are in order here. First, much of the surgery in medical potboilers and television dramas seems to be of this sort. In everyday life, when such dramatic surgery succeeds, it is often considered highly newsworthy, especially when the beneficiaries are young children. I suspect that if one were to take an index of articles in popular media about modern medical miracles, a greater proportion than one would expect by chance would be about pediatric patients—an indicator of how highly this society values youth.

Second, a question that I quite consistently and consciously bracketed during my field research was whether surgeons had met the demands of ethics and the law and obtained the "informed consent" of those patients for whom they wished to work miracles. I did not suspend judgment because I considered this problem unimportant. Quite to the contrary, it is one of the most complex and consequential questions one can ask about the delivery of care and the nature of professional-client relationships. I suspended judgment and bracketed the question because I was interested in surgeons' understandings of their social control responsibilities and in their definitions of error and failure. Whether the demands of "informed consent" were met or not was not a matter that surgeons considered a matter for social control. The quality of the consent obtained is not an issue that excites surgeons or affects their evaluation of each other. Moreover, I felt that acting as a conscience for my subjects and reminding them that "informed consent" was a matter that they should police would have been inappropriate; it would have made me a participant-advocate instead of a participant-observer.

I think that it is a sad commentary that in order to enter into the everyday world of surgeons one has to bracket such questions. However, it is also not clear whether a consideration of such matters would make surgeons any better or worse as surgeons. Here I apply the surgeon's own criteria of quality, which are clinical and narrow. Moreover, we might not be surprised that if the attending surgeon does not share his deliberations with his subordinates, he will not feel obligated to share them with his patients.

Further, there is in the very notion of "informed consent" as its definition has evolved a paradox that makes its achievement a virtual impossibility. To wit, to satisfy the demands of "informed consent," a surgeon, any physician, must, when suggesting a treatment to a patient, inform him of alternative treatments and their risks and benefits as compared to the proposed treatment. The patient's consent to treatment should ideally be free and not coerced. However, when the physician presents alternatives to the patient, he himself has already been persuaded of which alternative he prefers. So persuaded, it is hard to imagine that when he lays out to the patient his options, the physician does not order his discussion as a convincing argument for the alternative he favors and coerce the patient by his own belief in the correctness of his judgment. Hard to imagine because this is the way he has been taught to discourse on medical problems since his own training began.

In medicine, as opposed to sociology, making a diagnosis is not a value-free activity. Diagnosis is the rationale for intervention. It commits one to a course of action. Clinicians cannot leave the policy implications of their diagnoses for others to worry over. This is a luxury of sociologists and not of physicians in general or surgeons in particular.

Now, if the patient is informed of treatment plans by the physician's argument for what he thinks should be done, it is hard to conceive of truly informed consent for arguments themselves are structured by emphasizing some facts, minimizing some facts, and neglecting others entirely. If this is so, the physician's mode of discussion prevents him from laying out options in the impartial manner informed consent requires. Further, were he to do so, he might undermine the patient's trust and faith in his magical powers to cure—a trust and faith that medical anthropology informs us is an important part of the cure itself (Levi-Strauss 1963).

6. Unfortunately, I do not have data on the distribution of cases at Grand Rounds for the period of this study. However, the chief resident responsible for organizing the conference frequently voiced his concern to me that no service be underrepresented or overrepresented.

7. In the early days of open-heart surgery, there developed an interesting phenomenon known as the "Lazarus" syndrome, which is a corollary to patient presentation at rounds. Here, the surgeon waits in the recovery room with the patient and as he is coming out of anesthesia whispers in his ear: "You're alive. You're alive" (personal communication from David Schneider, Ph.D.). The syndrome is named for Lazarus rather than Christ, I imagine, more for the intensity of a patient's fear surrounding surgery, the awareness of the once-stopped heart beating again, and the patient's feeling that he has literally been raised from the dead than for the innate modesty and sense of propriety of cardiac surgeons. Patient presentation at Grand Rounds serves as evidence that all attendings have their Lazaruses and hence their opportunities to play Christ.

8. Coser (1961) and Hughes (1971) provide nice statements on how

guilty knowledge is shared by superordinates and subordinates. For all the protection attendings afford housestaff, they are given a great deal in return. In fact, a great danger to the professional whose activities are invisible to all but a handful of trusted subordinates is that a sharer of guilty knowledge will go public (see "Nurses Trigger Doctor Quiz," *Chicago Tribune*, 28 August 1974, p. 1). The codes of silence as they exist within licit and illicit occupations (see Maas 1968; Talese 1971) are a very revealing aspect of group life. The secret has received little attention since Simmel and deserves a great deal more. What people choose and work to keep unknown says much about them. The fit between the skeletons and the clothes in the closet is always of some interest and importance.

9. The retrospective peer-review conference conducted by the Department of Surgery differs considerably from the one conducted by the Department of Internal Medicine. In this latter conference, only one or two cases of interest are reported on. They are chosen for their heuristic value. They are intensively researched. Their presentation is separated from their occurrence by six to eight weeks. There is no attempt at this conference or elsewhere to make public and demand accounts for each death and complication that occurs as there is in the surgical conference. The public accounting of surgeons also differs considerably from what Light (1972) reports for psychiatrists.

Thus far, the literature on peer review has concentrated on the prospective review of clinical research (Gray 1975; Barber et al. 1973). These researchers conclude that such review improves the ethical performance of researchers, but how great such improvement is remains difficult to measure. The same problems exist for measuring the effectiveness of retrospective peer review. When questioned, all housestaff reported that one could and that they indeed did learn from the Mortality and Morbidity Conference. However, at the same time, they also expressed the belief that the best way to learn to manage complications was by actually managing them—an echo of the surgery-as-a-body-contact-sport philosophy.

10. This rule has an elastic quality about it; namely, the more minor the complication and the more happy the outcome, the more likely that the complication will be seen as "just one of those things," and the more likely that the subordinate will have complete accounting responsibility. In such cases the subordinate's original accounting to the attending is a dramatic rehearsal of the explanation he must later give in public.

11. An interesting feature of the presentation of such cases is that the recitation of a long list of injuries indicating a hopeless situation provokes anxious laughter among members of the audience.

12. The attending is obliged only by his own sense of his role and mission; he need not step forward, he may allow his subordinate to take the heat or he may absent himself entirely from the conference. Such a course of action is fraught with danger for attendings, however. I will discuss these dangers below.

13. The dynamics by which authority is undermined fall outside the already broad scope of this study. My impressions as far as attendings are concerned are sketchy since I was not so much an insider among them that attendings carried tales to me of each other's behavior. As far as subordinates are concerned, my impressions rest on a firmer basis. The housestaff on Baker accepted Arthur's authority despite his histrionics because they respected his integrity—it was a popular topic of conversation. On Able, where White and Peters were less open, authority was more subject to breakdown.

14. The concern with impression-management and saving face (Goffman 1967) has perhaps blinded us to the dynamics of altruistic sacrifice of face.

Chapter Five

1. This is not to say that no controls exist beyond this point but rather that this is the last institutionally structured one. Superordinates can drum offensive subordinates out of training at any point. However, the longer training continues, the greater is the burden of proof required to discredit an individual and thereby oust him. Second, the institutionalization of decision making can soften the blow for those who do not make the grade. The claim can legitimately be made that the decision is no reflection on them but testimony to how stiff the competition was that year. So, as a general rule, the longer one continues to train beyond the institutionalized decision-making point, the more difficult it is to separate him from the training program. This is a case of "If it were done when 'tis done, then 'twere well / It were done quickly" (*Macbeth*, act 1, scene 7).

2. Freidson and Rhea (1972) identify exclusion as the primary social control mechanism in a group practice. Freidson, in other writings (1970), identifies exclusion as the primary social control mechanism of

the medical profession. I extend these earlier discussions by showing the logic that physicians apply in deciding whom to exclude and whom to include.

3. Miller (1970) has borrowed Matza's (1964) concept of drift to explain the careers of interns in an elite training program. The term seems inappropriate for two reasons. First, a career in an elite institution requires the commitment of too much time and energy to be unthinkingly pursued. Second, superordinates play a too-important role in determining the currents subordinates are allowed to drift within. I think that in his interpretation Miller mistook what might have been a defensive rationalization subordinates used to soothe failure for a social process. Presumably people experience a great deal more difficulty than cream in drifting to the top.

4. Moreover, I suspect from my observations, but lack systematic evidence, that it is normative compliance rather than technical proficiency which leads attendings to choose subordinates as assistants on research. I expect a positive relationship between normative skills and sponsorship.

Chapter Six

1. Young physicians are taught techniques that encourage the patient to think he is "special" to the physician—always sit when visiting patients in their rooms, escort them from your clinic personally, develop a theme from their lives and structure discussion around it.

2. Retractors are known in the argot of surgery as "idiotsticks." The phrase conveys the degree of skill necessary to hold them properly. The maintenance of interest while standing at attention and keeping the patient's flesh clear of the operative field for hours on end is no easy task. However, superordinates take an inability to do this as an indication that an individual does not care about becoming a surgeon. Further, flagging interest insults the attending who is operating: he expects that his art will be appreciated for art's sake, if not merely for the utilitarian lessons a subordinate may learn.

Bibliography

Barber, Bernard; Lally, John J.; Makarushka, Julia Loughlin; and Sullivan, Daniel. *Research on Human Subjects: Problems of Social Control in Medical Experimentation.* New York: Russell Sage, 1973.

Becker, Howard. *Outsiders: Studies in the Sociology of Deviance.* New York: Free Press, 1963.

———. *Sociological Work: Method and Substance.* Chicago: Aldine, 1970.

Becker, Howard; Geer, Blanche; Hughes, Everett C.; and Strauss, Anselm. *Boys in White: Student Culture in Medical School.* Chicago: University of Chicago Press, 1961.

Bensman, Joseph, and Gerver, Israel. "Crime and Punishment in the Factory: The Function of Deviancy in Maintaining a Social System." *American Sociological Review* 28(1963):588–99.

Bittner, Egon. "The Police on Skid Row." *American Sociological Review* 32(1967a):239–58.

———. "Police Discretion in the Apprehension of Mentally Ill Persons." *Social Problems* 14(1967b):278–92.

Blum, Alan, and McHugh, Peter. "The Social Ascription of Motives." *American Sociological Review* 31(1971):98–109.

Bossert, Steven. "Tasks and Social Relationships in the Classroom." Ph.D. dissertation, University of Chicago, 1975.

Bucher, Rue. "Conflicts and Transformations of Identity: A Study of Medical Specialists." Ph.D. dissertation, University of Chicago, 1961.

Bucher, Rue, and Strauss, Anselm. "Professions in Process." *American Journal of Sociology* 66(1961):325–34.

Churchill, Lindsay. "Ethnomethodology and Measurement." *Social Forces* 50(1971):182–91.

Cicourel, Aaron. *The Social Organization of Juvenile Justice.*
New York: Wiley, 1969.

Cook, Robin. *The Year of the Intern.* New York: Signet Books,
1972.

Coser, Rose Laub. "Authority and Decision-Making in a Hospital." *American Sociological Review* 23(1958):56–63.

————. "Insulation from Observability and Types of Social
Control." *American Sociological Review* 26(1961):28–39.

Crane, Diana. *The Sanctity of Social Life.* New York: Russell
Sage, 1975.

Dalton, Melville. *Men Who Manage.* New York: John Wiley,
1959.

Daniels, Arlene K. "Military Psychiatry: The Emergence of a
Sub-specialty." In *Medical Men and Their Work*, edited by
Eliot Freidson and Judith Lorber. Chicago: Aldine-Atherton,
1972, pp. 145–62.

Daniels, Morris. "Affect and its Control in the Intern." *American Journal of Sociology* 66(1961):259–67.

Davis, Fred. "Uncertainty in Medical Diagnosis: Clinical and
Functional." *American Journal of Sociology* 66(1960):41–47.

Dewey, John. *Human Nature and Conduct.* New York: Modern
Library, 1922.

Emerson, Joan. "Behavior in Private Places: Sustaining Definitions of Reality in Gynecological Exams." In *Recent Sociology,
No. 2,* edited by Hans Dreitzel. New York: Macmillan, 1970,
pp. 73–97.

Erikson, K. T. *Wayward Puritans.* New York: John Wiley: 1966.

Foote, Nelson. "Identification as the Basis for a Theory of Motivation." *American Sociological Review* 16(1951):14–21.

Fox, Renée C. "Training for Uncertainty." In *The Student-Physician,* edited by Robert K. Merton, George Reader, and Patricia
Kendall. Cambridge: Harvard University Press, 1957*a*, pp.
207–41.

————. "The Autopsy: Its Place in the Attitude-Learning of
Second-Year Medical Students." Department of Sociology,
University of Pennsylvania, 1957*b*, unpublished.

————. *Experiment Perilous.* New York: Free Press, 1959.

———. "Ethical and Existential Developments in Contemporaneous American Medicine: Their Implications for Culture and Society." *Millbank Memorial Fund Quarterly*, Fall 1974, pp. 445–83.

Fox, Renée C., and Lief, Harold. "Training for 'Detached Concern' in Medical Students." In *The Psychological Basis of Medical Practice*, edited by Harold Lief, Victor Lief, and Nina Lief. New York: Harper and Row, 1963, pp. 12–35.

Freidson, Eliot. "Client Control and Medical Practice." *American Journal of Sociology* 65(1960):374–82.

———. *The Profession of Medicine: A Study in the Sociology of Applied Knowledge.* New York: Harper and Row, 1970a.

———. *Professional Dominance: The Social Structure of Medical Care.* New York: Atherton, 1970b.

———. *Doctoring Together.* New York: Elsevier, 1975.

Freidson, Eliot, and Rhea, Buford. "Processes of Control in a Company of Equals." In *Medical Men and Their Work*, edited by Eliot Freidson and Judith Lorber. Chicago: Aldine-Atherton, 1972, pp. 185–89.

Garfinkel, Harold. "Conditions of Successful Degradation Ceremonies." *American Journal of Sociology* 61(1956):420–24.

———. *Studies in Ethnomethodology.* Englewood Cliffs, N.J.: Prentice-Hall, 1967.

Glaser, Barney, and Strauss, Anselm. *The Discovery of Grounded Theory: Strategies for Qualitative Research.* Chicago: Aldine, 1967.

Glaser, Ronald J. *Ward 402.* New York: Braziller, 1973.

Goffman, Erving. *The Presentation of Self in Everyday Life.* Garden City, N.J.: Anchor-Doubleday, 1959.

———. *Encounters: Two Studies in the Sociology of Interaction.* Indianapolis: Bobbs-Merrill, 1961.

———. *Interaction Ritual: Essays on Face-to-Face Behavior.* Garden City, N.J.: Anchor-Doubleday, 1967.

———. *Relations in Public.* New York: Harper, 1971.

Goode, W. J. "Protection of the Inept." *American Sociological Review* 32(1967):5–19.

Goss, Mary E. W. "Influence and Authority among Physicians in an Outpatient Clinic." *American Sociological Review* 26(1961): 39-50.

Gray, Bradford H. *Human Subjects in Medical Experimentation.* New York: John Wiley, 1975.

Halberstam, David. *The Best and the Brightest.* New York: Fawcett, 1972.

Hughes, Everett C. *The Sociological Eye: Selected Papers on Work, Self, and Society.* Chicago: Aldine-Atherton, 1971.

Icheiser, Gustav. *Appearances and Realities.* San Francisco: Jossey-Bass, 1972.

Janowitz, Morris. *Social Control of the Welfare State.* Chicago: University of Chicago Press, 1976.

Levi-Strauss, Claude. *Structural Anthropology.* New York: Basic Books, 1963.

Lidz, Charles. "Rethinking Rapport: Problems of Reciprocal Obligations in Participant Observation Research." Paper presented at the annual meeting of the Eastern Sociological Association. New York, March 1977.

Light, Donald. "Psychiatry and Suicide: The Management of a Mistake." *American Journal of Sociology* 77(1972):821-38.

———. "The Sociological Calendar: An Analytic Tool." *American Journal of Sociology* 80(1975):1145-64.

Lukes, Steven. *Essays in Social Theory.* New York: Columbia University Press, 1977.

Lyman, Stanford, and Scott, Marvin. "Accounts." *American Sociological Review* 33(1968):46-62.

Maas, Peter. *The Valachi Papers.* New York: Putnam, 1968.

McHugh, Peter. *Defining the Situation.* Indianapolis: Bobbs-Merrill Co., 1968.

Matza, David. *Delinquency and Drift.* New York: John Wiley, 1964.

Mauss, Marcel. *The Gift.* New York: W. W. Norton, 1967.

Merton, Robert K. "Some Preliminaries to a Sociology of Medical Education." In *The Student-Physician,* edited by Robert K. Merton, George Reader, and Patricia Kendall. Cambridge: Harvard University Press, 1957, pp. 3-81.

Miller, Steven J. *Prescription for Leadership: Training for the Medical Elite.* Chicago: Aldine, 1970.

Mills, C. Wright. "Situated Actions and a Vocabulary of Motives." *American Sociological Review* 5(1944):904-13.

Mumford, Emily. *Interns: From Students to Physicians.* Cambridge: Harvard University Press, 1970.

Nolen, William J. *The Making of a Surgeon.* New York: Random
House, 1970.

————. *A Surgeon's World.* New York: Random House, 1972.

Parsons, Talcott. *Essays in Sociological Theory.* New York: Free
Press, 1949.

————. *The Social System.* New York: Free Press, 1951.

————. "Professions." In *The International Encyclopedia of the
Social Sciences.* New York: Macmillan, 1968, pp. 536-47.

Schwartz, Barry. "Waiting, Power, and Exchange: The Distribution of Time in Social Systems." *American Journal of Sociology* 79(1974):841-71.

Shils, Edward. *Center and Periphery: Essays in Macrosociology.*
Chicago: University of Chicago Press, 1975.

Siegler, Mark. "Pascal's Wager and the Hanging of Crepe." *New
England Journal of Medicine* 293(1975):853-57.

Simmel, Georg. *On Individuality and Social Forms,* edited by
Donald Levine. Chicago: University of Chicago Press, 1970.

Smelser, Neil J. *Theory of Collective Behavior.* London: Routledge & Kegan Paul, 1962.

Stelling, Joan, and Bucher, Rue. "Autonomy and Monitoring on
Hospital Wards." *Sociological Quarterly* 13(1972):431-47.

Sudnow, David. "Normal Crimes." *Social Problems* 12(1965):
255-76.

————. *Passing On: The Social Organization of Dying.* Englewood Cliffs, N.J.: Prentice-Hall, 1967.

————, ed. *Studies in Interaction.* New York: Free Press, 1972.

Sykes, Gresham, and Matza, David. "Techniques of Neutraliza-
tion: A Theory of Delinquency." *American Sociological Review*
22(1957):667-69.

Talese, Gay. *Honor Thy Father.* New York: World Publishers,
1971.

Viscott, David J. *The Making of a Psychiatrist.* New York: Arbor
House, 1974.

Webb, Eugene; Campbell, D. T.; Schwartz, R. D.; and Sechrest,

L. *Unobtrusive Measures: Nonreactive Research in the Social Sciences.* Chicago: Rand McNally, 1966.

Wender, Paul. "Vicious and Virtuous Circles: The Role of Deviation-Amplifying Feedback in the Origin and Perpetuation of Behavior." *Psychiatry* 31(1968):309–24.

X, Dr. *Intern.* New York: Harper and Row, 1965.

Zimmerman, Donald. "The Practicalities of Rule Use." In *Understanding Everyday Life,* edited by Jack Douglas. Chicago: Aldine, 1970, pp. 221–38.

Index

Able service, 8–11, 32, 69, 99, 103-4,
109, 197; attendings on, 10-11, 79,
81; authority on, 261; errors on, 13,
38–39, 41–42, 45–47, 52–54, 64;
exogenous failure on, 69; help
seeking on, 44; morale on, 207,
208; Mortality and Morbidity Conferences on, 145, 146; research
orientation of, 10, 11
Access to site, 194, 195
Accounts, 5, 31, 36, 98, 114, 255, 260;
and attendings, 96–97, 112–14;
relativity of, 30; responsibility and,
49, 50; strategies of, 129-30, 135-
36; and surgery, 30; types of, 141,
142; unnecessary, 120, 121. *See
also* Responsibility
Altruism, 261
American College of Surgeons, 58
Anesthesiologists, 105
Anonymity, 211, 212
Atherton, Bruce, x
Attendings, 3, 8–9, 11, 90, 123–24; and
accounts, 96–97, 113–14; as arbitrary, 89, 146; authority of, 84–86,
92, 113, 216; and competition, 150;
and conferences, 261; disagreements between, 9; discipline by, 84,
161; excuses and, 57–58, 76, 97-
98, 100; and fieldworker, 193–94,
197–98, 200-201; gatekeeping
function of, 148, 149; and housestaff, 37–38, 84; and judgmental
errors, 45, 48-49, 112; in Mortality
and Morbidity Conferences, 134-
36, 146; and normative errors,

53–55, 57–60; and quasi-normative
errors, 61–67; and residents, 158,
159; rounds of, 11–12, 79-84; and
students, 257; and technical errors,
37, 39, 112
Authority, 61, 201; attendings and,
84–86, 92; breakdown of, 261;
levels of, 9, 10; medical, 85; respect
for, 59; and scientific evidence, 86,
87; surgical, 65; undermining of,
261; Weber on, 113
Autonomy, zones of, 82
Autopsies, 174

Backstage, 112, 113; relativity of, 256
Baker service, 12–13, 32, 89, 91–94,
99-102, 105, 107, 109; attendings
on, 12–13, 79, 81, 83; chart rounds
on, 78; clinical experience on, 87,
88; decision making on, 96; expected failure on, 119, 120; Grand
Rounds on, 126, 127; judgmental
errors on, 49; Mortality and Morbidity Conferences on, 136-37,
145; normative errors on, 54–55,
59–60; quasi-normative errors on,
62–65, 67; scientific evidence
on, 86–89; technical errors on, 42-
43; work rounds on, 76
"Bandits," 187, 188
Barber, Bernard, 21, 188, 190, 255,
260, 263
Beatings, 6
Becker, Howard, 19–20, 205, 263
Bensman, Joseph, 263
Bershady, Harold, ix